PRAISE FOR

MW01097238

"*Rebel Mama* is a fun, relaxing read with a powerful underlying message. When you become a Rebel Mama, you realize you have the power to create your own birth experience. You don't need permission. You seek the support you need and you get to it.

Laura's personal style puts you at ease and delivers her message with authority and grace. Pregnant couples will enjoy every single page of this guide to creating the birth they want, navigating the system, and launching into parenthood whether you are having your first or your last baby.

Birth professionals would benefit, also, from taking notice of what families want. *Rebel Mama* is a five-star experience!"

~Barbara Harper,
RN, CLD, CCCE, Midwife, Founder/Director of Waterbirth International and author of *Gentle Birth Choices*

"With absolute honesty, exquisite perceptiveness, and a commitment to bury the concept of what is 'normal' for babies or parenting, Laura Rafferty (alias *Rebel Mama*) leaves absolutely nothing to the imagination and in so doing provides often a hilarious but remarkably comprehensive, edgy but always realistic and a warm-hearted picture of the magisterial highs and the inevitable challenges of becoming and being a mother. It is an intensely personal journey that she takes you on (no scientists needed here) an intensity that gives great vibrancy to the larger point she makes, and that is to trust yourself and your baby because there are as many ways to be that alleged elusive 'good mother' as there are mothers who strive to be one, that is, who strive and care to make their baby safe, secure and loved in whatever ways are possible, given her circumstances. I highly recommend the journey she will take you on."

~Dr. James McKenna,
Director of Mother Baby Behavioral Sleep Laboratory
at University of Notre Dame and author of *Safe Infant Sleep*

"*Rebel Mama* is a work of non-fiction in the memoir genre. It is suitable for the general reading audience and was penned by Laura Rafferty. The book follows the author's first year of motherhood in the middle of the Covid-19 pandemic. Upon deciding to have a child, the author realizes that in order to succeed and thrive in her new role she will need to abandon her previous approach of meticulously planning out her life and become a 'rebel mama.' This book is not intended to be a guide for new parents, but rather it is an opportunity for one new parent to share what helped her through the trials and tribulations of first-time parenthood.

This is a very candid sharing of a very personal experience in the author's life. The lockdowns around the globe that were initiated in response to the Covid-19 pandemic pushed people into situations that gave them a new perspective on their lives, and the idea of going through that experience whilst also becoming a parent for the first time boggles my mind with the emotional implications. Laura Rafferty, though, is a mother who learns to take life in her stride, and her skilled prose brings her journey alive with warmth and humor. *Rebel Mama* is a great read for first-time parents who are feeling overwhelmed. Not because it will provide them with step-by-step instructions on what to do but because it gives a feeling of solidarity for those parents who are overwhelmed by the process and are finding it hard to adapt to the new life with their child."

~Readers' Favorite,
ReadersFavorite.com

REBEL MAMA

*Breaking Free From Motherhood Norms and
Parenting From Within*

by

Laura Rafferty

Karen,
you are a veteran
rebel –thank you for
trailblazing

Laura Rafferty

To request permission, contact the publisher at rebelmamabook@gmail.com.

Paperback ISBN: 978-1-7376484-0-6
eBook ISBN: 978-1-7376484-1-3

First paperback edition: September 3, 2021

Edited by: Chantel Hamilton
Cover and Layout by: Sandy Kreps

Email: rebelmamabook@gmail.com

www.rebelmamawrites.com

Follow Laura on Instagram at @rebelmamawrites

CONTENTS

CONTENTS

To Jack,

Thank You.

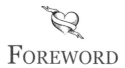

FOREWORD

As soon as you discover you are pregnant, you start "researching" (hello, Dr. Google), and when you share the happy news, you are bombarded with advice. It suddenly seems that everyone is an expert—on your baby!

Often, too, it seems that these experts offer a one-size-fits-all program of caring for babies—their way or the wrong way.

This book is different. Instead of advice, this is one real mother sharing her experiences of the conflict between her head and her powerful connection with her baby. Rebel Mama offers tips as she shares what worked for her, her partner, and her baby on the journey through a maze of popular advice that felt at odds with her instincts. However, she doesn't pretend to be an expert on anyone else's child.

The message is that you are the expert about your child. We all muddle through as we get to know this new little person, and it's OK to ditch advice that doesn't sit right for you and your baby.

Sadly, there is a conspiracy of silence around the struggles of new parents when your baby doesn't feed, sleep, or fit a convenient schedule. This isn't helpful and creates isolation as you wonder, Is there something wrong with our baby or are we doing something wrong?

Your baby isn't a tiny cardboard cut-out from the same template as your friends' baby. He is a unique little person, so of course he will respond differently. For instance, your baby's sleep needs will vary, just as our own needs vary from other adults', and we don't judge the adults who sleep the most as "good". In fact, we are more likely to call the sleepy ones "lazy sods," while those who need less sleep are now the "good" people.

Your baby's feeding needs will vary depending on his genetics— whether you are tall or short, solid or slightly built (you don't get rats from mice). If you are nursing, how often your baby needs to feed will also be influenced by your own breastmilk storage capacity. Think, some mamas have "shot glasses" while others have "jugs"! Although milk storage capacity isn't necessarily related to breast size (you can have small breasts with a good capacity of glandular tissue or larger breasts with less glandular tissue but more fat), obviously you will need far more "refills" if you have a "shot glass" milk storage capacity compared to a "schooner," as you need to get a certain volume into your baby over a day.

So how can we expect any one-size-fits-all schedule or program of advice to suit every baby?

It would be so much more helpful for all new parents, too, if there was more honesty about how hard it can be, how we all "stuff up" as we are faced with things like the reality of a newborn who doesn't appreciate our interior design skills (think fancy nursery) or the expensive gadgets that seemed so useful before we had an actual baby. Why won't he just rock off to sleep in that designer cot that cost more than your first car?

Rebel Mama is fun, funny, real, honest and non-judgy. However, among the messy and magical, it also contains evidence with references around contentious issues such as sleep and feeding.

This book will bust the conspiracy of silence around the new parent learning curve. Take from it what works for your own baby and your family. Remember, you are the expert on your own baby (and, of course, seek professional help if you are worried about your baby's health or development).

Above all, don't let anybody "should" on you, and if you feel confused about advice or it seems at odds with your intuition, try filtering it by asking yourself: Is it safe? Is it respectful? And, does it feel right?

~Pinky McKay,

IBCLC, bestselling author, TEDx speaker, mum of five, and no-rules nanny to four gorgeous grandkids.
www.pinkymckay.com

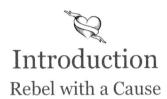

Introduction
Rebel with a Cause

I never had the chance to go to rehab or therapy. Let's be honest, I barely had the chance to go to the bathroom in peace. I didn't get the chance to ease my way out of old habits or lie on the office couch of a stranger with a psychology degree diploma on the wall above me, working through what it all meant. There was no 28-day rehab nor 12-step program. I went cold turkey, ripped the Band-Aid off.

This book is my recovery. This book helped me sort out my transformation. This book gave me an outlet to make sense of it all and put my journey into words. And, it is my gift to every new mama, or expecting mama, who needs some inspiration to awaken her rebellious side and storm the gates of modern parenting practices.

Hi, my name is Laura, and I'm a recovering rule-aholic.

I've loved rules and structure, and for as long as I can remember, I've been easily annoyed by anyone who can't follow protocol. I once got into a full-blown fight with my husband, followed by a period of silent treatment, because we were doing a thirty-day clean eating cleanse and he cheated one day by eating French fries and having a beer. I couldn't comprehend and was disheartened that he couldn't stick to the rules. Thankfully we got over that hump because he was an integral part in the baby-making process.

I pride myself on doing the right thing. I made my younger sister a WWLD (What would Laura do?) charm bracelet to wear on her wrist at all times when she studied abroad for a semester in college in London. Rules, in her mind, are loose guidelines, and I was petrified she'd get herself into trouble having too much fun under Big Ben's watch.

I wasn't just a rule-aholic, I've also always been a plan-aholic. Need a well laid out plan? Need a strategy on how to accomplish a new undertaking? Looking for someone to guide the way? Let's go, I'm ready. I organize the trips, I plan the parties, I map out the adventures. A few of my closest friends tagged me with the classy HBIC nickname (Head Bitch in Charge, in case you run with a more sophisticated crew) when that became a thing back in the 2000s.

I don't have the words to underscore this anal-retentive nature of mine. We're talking spreadsheets are my happy place. To-do lists and Post-it notes make me smile. Bring me chaos, and I will transform it into order like a magician with a wand. I spent over ten years climbing the corporate ladder, leapfrogging peers and superiors because I operate in a get-shit-done kind of way. I've been called a robot, a machine, and half-human many times, and I assumed I'd plow through motherhood in a similar fashion.

This isn't just an adulthood trait either. I'm pretty sure I've been this way my entire life, although my memory before age five is foggy, and my parents are too biased to weigh in. But, I never sat in time out. I was never sent home with a poor report card. I was raised Roman Catholic and my holy-rolling eight-year-old self was grateful to Moses for putting stone to tablet, giving us the guidelines for life. And a dialogue like...

"We can't go in the pool yet; it hasn't been thirty minutes since we ate lunch," eleven-year-old me said to my nine-year-old sister.

"Who cares? Mom can't see us," she replied.

"But, Marissa, that's the rule!"

...is just one of countless conversations tweenage me had with my younger sister about doing what we're told.

Fast forward twenty years from that day at the pool, when I became pregnant, and naturally I had full intentions of following all of the parenting rules set forth by today's pediatric experts.

√ Labor: When the time comes to birth baby, follow the lead of the nurses and doctors.

√ Circumcision: If baby is a "he", then I will get him circumcised.

√ Sleep:

- When it comes to sleep, baby will sleep separately in a bassinet, on their back.

- Baby will be put down awake but drowsy, so they learn to fall asleep by themselves.

√ Breastfeeding:

> • When it's time to feed, I will only nurse baby every two to three hours.

> • And speaking of nursing, I will do so until he/she is twelve months old, and then wean.

√ Real Food: Solid foods will be introduced in the form of purées starting at six months.

√ Child Care: When it comes to being a working mom, I will take my sixteen-week maternity leave and then arrange appropriate childcare.

√ Mom Guilt: I'll be separated from my baby ten plus hours per day, five days per week, guilt-free.

√ Perfection: Of course, I'll be sure to do it all with a smile, documenting the entire first year with fancy photos and ending it with a big bang first birthday party.

I love a solid plan, and it sounded straight-forward to me. Quite frankly it didn't even seem that hard. I had plenty of friends who had done it, and figured if they could, so could I. I was good to go, ready to do this motherhood thing.

But, as my bump grew, so did my doubts. Not my doubts in my ability to be a good mom, but my doubts in these so-called rules. The further I dug, none of those standards were making sense. I was finding that maybe what looked good on paper didn't really hold true in practice. Slowly, I was starting to feel that the guidance given to pregnant women and new moms was in direct conflict to what my gut was telling me to do. By the time I was ready to give birth, I had subscribed to the theory that rules were meant to be broken. By the time my son, Jack, celebrated his first birthday, I had completely transformed from rule-following soon-to-be mama to rebel mama.

I can remember driving to Jack's six-month doctor appointment saying to my husband, Justin, "You know the drill. He only nurses every two to three hours during the day; and yes he sleeps in our room, but he sleeps by himself in the bassinet." We were prepping our lies for the doctor, the guy we're supposed to rely on for sound parenting advice. What was wrong with me?! I'm an adult, goddamn it. I have a big-girl job, pay big-girl bills, yet all of a sudden I'm acting like a little girl hiding the truth from her parents! None of it felt right.

Shortly after that doctor appointment, something completely unimaginable happened. Something that was crippling to many, but by some bizarre twist of fate, was a game changer for me as a new mom. COVID-19 was born, a pandemic hit the world, and I found myself home around the clock just a few short months after I had returned to the office from maternity leave. While I was still working at home, the separation I previously had from my baby was swapped with separation from society. This separation allowed me to further let go of social norms and mother from my heart. I had the unique opportunity to mother like no one was watching. (In the right kind of way, not in the "call social services on that crazy lady" kind of way.)

The pandemic not only required us to be in isolation, but it required us to make a mentality shift. A completely different and foreign way of viewing life, one that you could have never predicted. Normal had to be redefined. Routines had to be adjusted. Much of the same could be said about what motherhood requires of us. It doesn't matter how well you plan, curve balls come your way. So, while the world was busy writing new rules, I was busy breaking old ones. Safety, structure, and strict guidelines were the focus of everyone during COVID-19, and I was basically throwing the rule books out the window. Not unlike the world after the pandemic, I'll never be the same; nor will I ever forget this transformation, forever imprinted by the transition to motherhood.

COVID-19 allowed me to mother with very little opportunity for judgement, a rare gift in this day and age. Being a mom can be so hard if we let it be, and when we let ourselves be susceptible to the judgement of others, it feels even harder. I've often contemplated why is there so much judging of new moms? I've decided that it's because being a parent challenges you in SO MANY WAYS, makes you so uncomfortable and uncertain in your decisions at times (or at all times), and no one wants to think they did it wrong or screwed up.

It might not feel good for a woman to watch her daughter breastfeed her grandbaby until age two when she herself gave up after a couple weeks and fed her daughter formula. She may feel like a failure and that she messed up and did her daughter wrong. Or even worse, she could be too narrow-minded to think there was a different (dare I say more optimal?) way to do things. So she stubbornly believes her daughter is "ruining" or "spoiling" her grandbaby. There's a better way to look at it though. One of my favorites quotes to live by is from Maya

Angelou: "Do the best you can until you know better. Then when you know better, do better."

With regards to messing up this parenting thing, I've got good news and bad news for all the mamas out there. Let's start with the bad news: You will absolutely screw it up at some point along the way. It's inevitable, the concept of super mom is just as fictitious as Wonder Woman. The good news? You won't screw it ALL up. Seriously, even if you really, really suck, you successfully grew and birthed that little human which means...cut yourself some slack, you've done some things well.

I doubt you really suck, even if that's what you've been telling yourself. My guess is you probably picked up this book because you needed someone to tell you it's okay to listen to your gut and not mainstream media. If you were truly happy with the way things were going for you, then this book might not have been on your radar. I mean truly happy, as in comfortable and at peace with your decisions, not happy as in pleased with the perception others have of you as a mother. Herein lies my attempt at encouraging you to be a rebel, screw all the advice and rules and get in tune with your inner mama because only she knows what's best for you and your family.

Eleanor Roosevelt nailed it when she said, "Do what you feel in your heart to be right, for you'll be criticized anyway. You'll be damned if you do and damned if you don't." (Yes, I will be quoting all the inspirational role models of the world throughout this book, so get used to it now. Grab a notebook, write them down; they're gems to live by.) Typically, I don't enjoy confrontation, and I like making people happy. I'm generally a pleasant person (if I do say so myself). I don't like criticism that doesn't come in the form of constructive criticism (and oftentimes that doesn't even feel so good). Because of those personality traits, I've gone along with the crowd on mothering sagas more times than I am pleased to admit, regardless if I agree or not, so as to not create waves in the dialogue or be viewed as weird or different. To be honest, sometimes I've gone along with the crowd because the thought of having to educate and enlighten others on a different way of thinking can feel so daunting to a mama who is already drained as it is!

Mamas, we need to stop that. We've created this ridiculous culture of always feeling the need to be able to relate to each other with the intention of fitting in or conforming to the norm. Everyone and their brother are on social media trying to be relatable. What happened to different strokes for different folks? I spent enough years in a corporate job having the power of diversity drilled in my head. You don't want to be surrounded by a bunch of you's to achieve the best outcome. You want to be surrounded by a diverse group of individuals to get different perspectives and ideas to have your mind opened to other possibilities than the reality in which you know.

We don't question enough of what we do, numbed by following the crowd and consumed with what others will think of us. We're all too programmed, too robotic. In a fascinating study on authoritative knowledge, fear appeals are often used to influence our attitudes and behaviors[1] , resulting in us abandoning faith in our natural abilities.

We forget that we are a species of mammals, and we've lasted this long as a species because of our survival instincts. Evolution has most certainly changed us over time, but at our core we are far more like our ancestors from hundreds of thousands of years ago than we are not.

Have you ever stopped and thought about why women have boobs, or am I the only one who contemplates the wonders of the world? Well, let me tell you where I landed on this mind-bender. Women have breasts for the sole purpose of producing and providing milk to their offspring. Believe it or not, the ta-tas are not part of the female physique to keep lingerie companies in business nor to lure men into buying us a drink. We were literally made to nourish our babies. It's completely natural and all part of the circle of life. It sounds simple and fundamental, yet breastfeeding is just now becoming normalized, and even so, it still has its cynics who claim it's gross or unnecessary thanks to the "convenience" of formula.

Let me tell you, there is nothing convenient about motherhood (except you finally now have an excuse to say "no" to the neighbor who keeps asking you to attend her Pampered Chef party). If you were looking for a whole lot of cuteness in your life with minimal effort, you probably should have bought a goldfish.

The lure of convenience has gotten out of control. Sure, the washing machine and microwave helped save time for the 1950s housewife, but options like formula and sleep training are convenience temptresses to the exhausted and overwhelmed mama. So many "solutions" surround us; but what we sometimes don't realize is solutions imply there is a problem, but maybe the only problem is our perspective?

It's time we allow ourselves to get back to basics, tune out the outside world and tune in to ourselves. Throwing a pandemic in the mix of new motherhood helped to quiet the societal influence of family and friends and allowed me to mother from within and without judgement, boycotting these social norms. In addition, being quarantined provided an opportunity to slow down life, making these conveniences in parenthood less urgent.

Somewhere someone said the days feel long but the years they fly. There will be so many hard, trying, throw-in-the-towel, stick-a-fork-in-me moments where some of the convenient solutions are going to seem ideal. The reality is, though, you'll blink, and these moments will be over; and you'll miss them more than you ever knew you could miss a moment.

There is no sugar-coating it. Becoming a mama will shake you to your core, make you dig deep and find out who you really are and then transform you into that person. She may look very different than the woman you were when you got pregnant. The transformation is terrifying, enlightening, invigorating, a complete white-knuckler. It's literally like a trip on the Tower of Terror amusement park ride.

You have two options. You can squeeze your eyes shut and hold on for dear life and pray like hell it's over faster than it started. Or, you can throw your hands in the air, scream with joy, and feel the biggest rush of your life. Either way, you're going to be on one of the biggest free falls of your life.

I won't undermine the fact that it's confusing and overwhelming to navigate all the information out there. I get it. I've read some dry, painstaking literature and information available on all the topics I discuss in here. I've sifted through all the propaganda and manipulation to try to find some version of the truth that resonated with me. I became obsessive the more I learned and the more I uncovered. My house was covered in books on baby sleep, breastfeeding, attachment parenting, and baby-led weaning: terms and words I didn't even know existed back when I peed on that stick. My eyes were opened wider and wider, and I felt more and more validated with the turn of every page, oftentimes mouth agape at how ill-advised we all are as new moms. After digging into many of the topics with hours of research, I validated my gut reactions, both disturbing me and saddening me that there is so much misguidance out there shared with women during an already tumultuous time. While I'll tell you more than once to follow your gut, for me it was super helpful to understand the biology and/or psychology behind many of these topics. I have a logic-loving brain, and I needed to organize the information in a sensical way.

Here's one to whet your palate: Do you know that babies are born with a brain that is only 25% that of which it will be by adulthood.[2] It's a fascinating story. Ever since we became a bipedal mammal millions of years ago (i.e. we walk on two legs instead of four), a mother's hips, pelvis, and groin are now only so wide. Therefore, the baby has to come out before the brain (and ultimately the head) is too big to fit through the exit door[3] (although I will argue that thanks to the Shakira hips I was gifted, I probably could have birthed a baby whose brain was at least 1/3 of what it would be by adulthood).

Which parts the brain are developed and good to go versus still needing to be formed? Yep, you guessed it. Babies' brain stems are ready for action when they're born. That's the part responsible for blinking, pooping, breathing, etc.—the unconscious functions, the ones we need for survival. The rest of the brain, including the cerebellum and cerebrum, still have some cooking to do, which is why a baby doesn't come out walking, talking, and feeding himself with a fork.[4] And, he certainly doesn't come out with the ability to decipher emotions or solve a sudoku puzzle. Here's the part that really wowed me: The brain isn't fully developed until age 25![5] This might explain some of your decisions in college.

So, the whole "he's manipulating you, you don't have to answer his every whimper" or "teach baby to self soothe so he sleeps through the night" is nothing but a bunch of hocus pocus. Baby is literally unable to manipulate or self soothe—both of those come later in life (enter, the teenage years).

Repeat after me: The baby brain is not a miniature adult brain. Yes, the baby foot is a miniature adult foot (and the cutest thing ever), so it's hard for us to comprehend how the brain isn't the same. In reality, it is undeveloped and cannot understand the things we're hoping like hell it can (like go the bleep to sleep or play by yourself for five flipping minutes so mommy can pour a cup of much needed coffee). Teaching a baby independence isn't a thing, and while being independent has its place in life, that place is not the nursery.

How I Organized This Book

Look, I'm a recovering rule-aholic, but I still enjoy structure where structure makes sense, okay? So, I did you a solid and organized this book in a way that allows for easy navigation. (You get enough practice with difficult navigation making your way through motherhood!)

Each chapter is broken down into three sections:

1. *Road to Rebellion*—This is where I open my heart and soul to you (and sometimes my bra and legs too). The humbling and eye-opening experience of raising my sweet baby boy inspired me to share all these fumbles and findings. I tell my story not because I claim to be accredited, an expert, or a doctor. I'm just a new mom to my baby boy who keeps me on my toes and a loving wife to a husband I drive completely bananas. I love them so much and my main goal in life is to give them a good life. Know that these are purely my experiences and opinions, with a little bit of research and a whole lot of gut feeling (a lost art in my opinion). I tell them to you, though, because my gut (see, there it goes again) says I can't possibly be alone; and even if there is just one ounce of reservation in you, questioning what I questioned or doubting what I doubted, read on.

2. *Redefining Normal*—This is where gut feeling meets data, and I redefine normal. We're going to totally geek out on the evidence that backs up our maternal instincts. It is nearly impossible that every new mom will have a global pandemic allowing her to mother from within, literally and figuratively, so leverage my findings to help you find your way. My objective is to make you aware that what is dubbed as normal might not be that normal at all. Spoiler alert: I am a total nerd. We're talking Coke-bottle glasses and all. (Thank goodness for contact lenses, for without them my high school life might have been a challenge). While I enjoyed much of the research,

I recognize not everyone might find it so enjoyable. In fact, many would probably find it pretty overwhelming, but I find that fact checking your gut, ah, is so validating. Therefore, I tried to boil all of this down to the information that made an impact on me and factored into my decision making (or in some cases the data that just totally blew my mind and it didn't feel right to keep to myself) and present it in a way that's easy and enjoyable to consume. I did this because you're busy and because so much of the material out there is dense, dull, and oftentimes a little too hippy or crunchy granola, which turns off some people. Please don't mistake any of this as me justifying all my parenting decisions to the world. I'm not trying to rationalize the choices I've made or the way I do motherhood. Quite the opposite; I couldn't care less who's on board with me, hence the rebel part. It's not justification nor rationalization, it's revelation.

3. *What Worked for Me*—This is not advice. I repeat, this is not advice. This is me telling you how I adjusted from what I thought I was supposed to do to what I ended up doing. This is intended to inspire you to forge your own road to rebellion. My story is not your story. This is not one of those how-to guides, nor is my journey an instruction manual for you. While difficult to admit for someone like me, there is no structure, nor order, in which we can prescribe how one should handle motherhood. Instead, I hope to awaken you, make you come alive, and feel comfortable challenging the norm, rebelling against the masses, as you walk away from these pages, feeling more educated and empowered. I basically put my diary out there for the world in hopes I can stir inside you what's been stirred inside me. To give you the confidence that I had to find in myself. To share with you the facts and how they've influenced my story. Research was my medicine; writing was

my therapy. You know they say dance like no one is watching? I want you to mama like no one is watching. It's going to be uncomfortable and clunky and you'll oftentimes feel like you have two left feet; but your baby will think you're a world-class ballerina, and you'll eventually find your footing. You'll live with no regrets, and you will raise a confident, secure, and happy little baby.

You'll also find some bonus material, my *Secret Weapons*, sprinkled throughout the book. These items were my go-to's and helped me combat my journey into motherhood and through baby's first year.

Finally, I've written this topically such that each reader can choose how they want to tackle it. Devour it like an ice cream sundae all in one sitting or ration it like imported chocolates. Some people have a hefty appetite and the capacity to take it all in at once. Others need to digest piece by piece; it's a lot to absorb! Skip the chapters that's don't pertain to you (Having a girl? You may not care about circumcision.) or bounce around to where you're most interested. This book is not always sequential. Sometimes Jack is three days old and sometimes he's eight months. So, keep up! No dozing off!

LET'S PLAY NICE IN THE SANDBOX

Does it sound a little like I'm setting up running rules for how to approach this book? Did I mention I'm still recovering? But real talk, let's practice what we preach to our little ones and play nice in the sandbox together.

Listen, there are many of you who won't like what you read. In fact, things might even get uncomfortable at times. I bet some of you have already gotten defensive in what you've read thus far. I'm discussing some pretty controversial topics, of which have severed friendships, relationships, and even marriages for many mamas who took the rebel road (not unlike how different folks managed COVID-19 rules and regulations and the strain that put on many relationships). Personally, while I haven't experienced anything to this extreme, I have naturally found myself distancing from (perhaps even avoiding) friends and relations whom I know do not agree with some of my decisions. I did find myself incredibly hurt and frustrated when loved ones would make a joke like, "What will happen sooner? He'll go to kindergarten or he'll sleep in his own bed?" Or ask, "How long are we going to do this for?" while I was nursing him.

If these topics can tear apart well-rooted relations, I'm not expecting our relationship that we just started a few pages ago to necessarily survive. It would be cool if we could agree that even though we may have differing opinions, it doesn't make either of us wrong. That's just the point! I'm sharing with you because I want you to know it's OKAY to not be a follower if you don't want to be. You don't have to follow me or any other mama. Create your own path through motherhood, and find confidence in your abilities along the way. You will build knowledge, and knowledge builds confidence, and confidence builds a strong mom who responds to her baby's needs and tells everyone else to go scratch if they have a different opinion.

Treat this book like the warm hug and the belly laugh every mom needs in the first year of motherhood (Because who doesn't love laughing? I would consider it one of my top pastimes.), not the judgmental look nor the raised eyebrow nor the shaking of the head in disapproval so many of us receive. There is no perfect or right or normal when it comes to parenting; those words are all made up, based on perception and not reality. I'm not debunking myths. I'm telling you why I broke the rules. Some of these rules might work fantastically for you and your baby, and that's super. Really, I'm happy for you. We need to be supportive of each other, regardless of our choices.

I am also not shaming the other side, but we've become too censored to the point that what we're saying says nothing at all, such as "Circumcise or don't circumcise, the pros and cons are basically equal." Gee, thank you, SUPER helpful. Or, we're so conservative that our advice is contradictory when looked at holistically, such as "Hey, be sure you have lots and lots of skin-to-skin with baby, but DO NOT sleep with baby." Wait, what? My intent is not to offend, my intent is to inform.

I'm not encouraging you to start a debate or argument with every parent you don't see eye-to-eye with because that's not going to make things any better. What we need to commit to is trying to find our voice and share our true thoughts and feelings in the right moments, or none of these topics will ever be better understood and considered.

Play this one out for me. When talking to a fellow mama about baby sleeping, what if you didn't say, "Ugh, I totally hear you. Listening to them cry it out is the worst," and instead said, "I haven't let him cry it out. Instead, he sleeps with us, and all three of us are getting great sleep now," and you open that other mama's eyes to another option, one she didn't even consider because it had been touted as taboo? I think you'll be pleasantly surprised at the influence you could have when you stay true to yourself when talking with others.

Snuggle in, Mama. Grab your tea or coffee (Hell, grab your wine. It's a judgement-free zone, after all.), and sit back and relax. I'm thrilled you're here, and I'm honored to take you through how I broke my rule-following addiction. Let's talk vaginas, penises, breasts, tongues, and more. While right now that may now sound a little bit like either a boring anatomy class or a cheesy Harlequin novel, I promise you it will turn out to be way more than such for you. Keep reading if you're ready to find out how raising a baby (during a global pandemic to boot) allowed me to listen to my inner mama and rebel against modern maternal norms.

THE WHOLE IS GREATER THAN
THE SUM OF ITS PARTS

I feel like you should know a little bit more about me since we're about to get intimately down and dirty. And, by a little bit more about me, I mean you should be aware of my viewpoint on how I approach every aspect of life.

While this book is about entering motherhood and caring for your tiny human, I'd be remiss if I didn't acknowledge that is only one part of who you are as a person. You must not lose sight of the fact that you are a human being who must eat, drink, sleep, breathe, and if you're lucky, love and be happy. Read: You have needs that must be met in order to have any chance of being successful as a mama.

So, Mama, listen up. You can follow your gut and be a rebel parent with me, but you are useless if you're only taking care of your mom parts and not your whole being (figuratively and literally). You need to eat well (Think of Michael Pollan's simple advice to eat food, not too much, mostly plants.), move your body, make sure you're at an optimal weight for performance (I did not just say a size zero, I said a weight that makes it so you feel good and can move and groove—be realistic about your body.), sleep whenever you can, and get outside as often as you can. And for the love of all things good, lighten up and have fun; laughter is good for the soul.

You need a support system in place. This mommy thing takes a village, yet ironically so many women often feel very alone in those early days of motherhood. That doesn't always mean you have sixteen cousins and aunts and siblings in a constant rotation helping you. (But, man, wouldn't that be nice? I always envy those women.) You can have a friend on text message standby whom you can ask for advice or whine about your day. Go online and find a La Leche League leader or group near you. Just find some network where you're not isolated and where you have a place to go when YOU need an outlet. A spouse or partner is an ideal place to start, but I recognize not everyone has one of those, or even if you do, they might suck (keeping it real, my friends).

Hey! Snap out of it, did you just gloss over those last few paragraphs? Take your eyes back up there and read it again.

Then, always remember this little parable. My husband is a big podcast guy. He listens to them all the time, and so I indirectly listen to them when he tells me the latest nugget he's learned. One day he tells me how good blueberries are for you, and how some guy ate a cup of blueberries every day. (I'm sure it was some very influential dude, but I don't remember who.) I said, "Well, that's great, but does he also have high blood pressure? And smoke cigars? And cheat on his wife? Because if the answer is yes to any of the above, his eight-ounce serving of blueberries isn't doing a thing for him." I was being dramatic, yes, but I was doing so to make a point. I'm a firm believer in looking at things holistically and not in silos.

I approach life much like I've approached this first year of motherhood—ensuring that my individual actions and decisions are all pointing in the same direction. As I mentioned, that direction might not be the exact same direction as you're pointing. The key is that we're all following our own true north and staying in harmony with ourselves.

Speaking of harmony within oneself, let's talk about your endocrine system and how one of my favorite parts of motherhood is getting high. Okay, go ahead, call my bluff. I might have become a rebel mama, but I still remained a square in some areas. You're right, I'm not talking Bob Marley's kind of "high" here, but I am talking a euphoric high that your body creates all its own from two of the coolest mama hormones ever.

The first is prolactin, the hormone of mothering. Yes, there is literally a hormone responsible for that so called "maternal instinct" that many mamas have, and it goes by the name of prolactin.[6] Prolactin helps mamas fall in love with their baby immediately. Understanding its existence completely demystified for me how moms of ugly babies think their baby is the most adorable thing in the world. Furthermore, prolactin is responsible for milk production, and so women who breastfeed naturally have an easier time finding patience for their baby during trying times[7] (like every damn meal time) thanks to the good vibes it gives us. Prolactin is also found in breastmilk and is optimal for brain development.[8] Since we know babies' brains take years to fully grow, this furthers the case for extended breastfeeding.

The other endocrine wonder is oxytocin. This little gem is responsible for helping the uterus contract and push out the baby during labor. It is also the hormone behind our milk let down when nursing.[9] (I see a theme here—oxytocin is a pusher of all the goods.) It is known as the hormone of love and is released when we have an orgasm but also with simple gestures of affection such as touching, hugging, or even sharing a meal.[10]

Both hormones can help mamas relax, even make them sleepy. Dr. Sarah Buckley shares, "After a nursing episode, breastfeeding mothers are calmer, with an elevation in mood and increased resistance to stress: these effects are likely to be due to the peaks of oxytocin and prolactin, both stress-reducing hormones."[11] Stress-reducing hormones? Yes, please!

If we just get out of our own way, take a back seat and let our bodies and our babies take over, more often than not things will operate like a well-oiled, harmonious machine. I'm calling in these two friends to prove it to you, oxytocin and prolactin.

If we choose a drug-free labor, oxytocin will help push out the baby and give us all the good feels about our baby. Prolactin will be in full swing, and our milk will come in. If we skip the circumcision, there's a greater chance of baby latching and prolactin to keep doing its thing. Bed sharing, to nurse around the clock and keep our milk supply up, helps baby and mommy to sleep and comforts during physical and mental developmental milestones (teething or separation anxiety, anyone?). And finally, those stress-relieving vibes calm the pressures of mom guilt and perfection.

This is not witchcraft. I didn't imagine or dream up these ways. God, I sure did feel crazy at times along the way, but awareness of these two hormones reminded me that it's TOTALLY BIOLOGICALLY NORMAL and to kindly please sit the hell down and let them do their thing. Let's link arms with prolactin and oxytocin as we skip down my road to rebellion.

1

Bumpy Trip to the Bump
Conception

ROAD TO REBELLION

My baby was no "oops". Getting pregnant took over a year, thanks to some stubborn reproductive parts of mine. (Let the record show, Justin's sperm were on point.)

Like many pre-motherhood sexually-active women, I had been on birth control for the better part of my adult life. Some say that's promiscuous; others say it's precautionary. Either way you view it, I knew that it was time to say goodbye to that tiny pencil eraser-sized pill if I wanted to become a mama. What I didn't know was that I would have to do much more than just stop swallowing a pill daily in order to get pregnant.

I waited a few months for my period to return, as I was aware it often took up to three months to get your cycle back on track. Because I wasn't getting a period during that time, I had no idea when I could possibly be ovulating and ultimately getting pregnant. So, I bought several pregnancy tests. We're talking an embarrassing amount of pregnancy tests. Speaking of embarrassing, I was so uninformed at the beginning of this journey that I was taking pregnancy tests the day after we'd have sex, thinking that they were that fast in identifying the pregnancy hormones in your urine stream. It's okay if you're laughing at me, or possibly laughing with me, because you did the same. Turns out, it takes at least two weeks before any trace of the pregnancy hormones is detectable in your urine. Also, my doctor shared with me that it can take up to a week for the impregnated egg to attach itself to your uterine wall. So, while the sperm joins with the egg within a couple of days of having sex (Even THAT isn't instantaneous.), it's a bit of time before your whole body realizes it has company.

Three months came and went with no visit from Aunt Flow, and I decided in an attempt not to waste more time (and not waste any more money on pregnancy tests), I'd go see the doctor. After my first ever internal ultrasound (Am I the only one who sees nothing but a curling iron when they take out that device?), I was diagnosed with Polycystic Ovarian Syndrome (PCOS)—an acronym I had never heard of before. I was told I had little tiny cysts all over my ovaries prohibiting me (or at least making it more difficult than normal) from ovulating and ultimately getting a period.

FABULOUS. Just what I wanted to hear when trying to conceive. In typical Laura fashion, I dove right into how we get rid of these pesty little cysts so we can get back in business. My doctors responded by immediately rattling off a timeline for a prescription program, first starting with a dose of progesterone and then a round of Clomid. The plan was that the synthetic progesterone would force my uterus lining to shed, and the Clomid (an infertility drug they give to women to jump-start ovulation) would initiate a cycle. All I could picture were little elves taking defibrillator paddles to my ovaries. Between each of these treatments, I'd have regular dates with the vagina curling iron and the blood lab so that they could monitor the activity in my ovaries and the hormone levels in my blood at various points in time. All of this was to occur within one menstrual cycle— essentially, I was signing up for a month of being a lab rat.

Okay, so this wasn't exactly how I anticipated things to go, but these are the experts, so I had to get on board, right? It was a fun couple of weeks, bouncing between popping progesterone and Clomid pills, having blood work drawn, and staring at my underwear every time I went to the bathroom, trying to manifest a red stain.

I wore a chastity belt and all and avoided Justin while taking Clomid because the doctor warned it could increase my chance of having twins. Of course, I wanted to get pregnant, but I was not mentally ready for twins. To all my twin mamas out there, I know that no one is ever really ready for that BOGO. At this point in the infertility journey, I was hoping to use Clomid for the sole purpose of "jump starting my cycle".

I did the blood work, I had the internal ultrasound, and I got nothing but disappointing news. I didn't release an egg. The internal ultrasound is used to measure the size of the maturing eggs in my ovaries. According to the ultrasound tech, in order for an egg to "drop", it needs to grow to about 1.8 – 2.8 centimeters. My largest one was barely 1 centimeter. Optimistic that maybe this runt could still take the fallopian tube journey, the deal was sealed when my blood work was taken and there was no spike in the hormones that would usually spike if an egg were released. It was a great attempt, but a fail nevertheless.

I could do Clomid two more times before we started looking at IVF and IUF. The doctor was still hopeful because the first time around he prescribed me the lowest possible dose of Clomid, so he felt by increasing the dosage, I'd have a better chance.

Because of the need for all the monitoring and charting and timing, we took a month off before doing it all over again. I was super busy with a new project at work and traveling all the time. My schedule was not going to allow for the multiple trips to the doctor's office and blood lab, not to mention finding time to smooch my husband. Two months after the first act, I was finally able to squeeze in another few weeks of this madness amongst work travel, and we tried again. This time I said the hell with it, there must be some truth behind Double Mint gum's "double your fun" jingle. Let's go for twins! Chastity belt removed, Clomid dosage jacked up, we did it again. The only thing that doubled was our disappointment.

Deflated, stressed, and emotionally drained, I said I needed some time before trying again. I knew we only had one more round of Clomid before I'd have to go into a world of infertility treatments that I wasn't even close to being prepared to enter.

Truthfully, I wasn't prepared even for the Clomid experiments. All the drugs and monitoring went against my holistic all-natural mantra, and I just needed to take five. It was an abundance of fake hormones and chemicals pumped into me in a short period of time. Looking back, I realize that pause was my first act of rebellion. Rebellion doesn't always come in the form of guns blazing, but I listened to my gut and gave myself the space to absorb all that had happened and took time to think through how I wanted to proceed.

We carried on with life, trying to ignore this nagging concern that infertility was knocking on our door. I had weeks of international travel ahead of me, and we decided that when that settled down and I was home long enough to make a baby, we'd pick up where we left off.

Part of me was grateful for the break, because you know what they say, "A watched pot never boils." The other part of me was worried we were delaying the inevitable. However, off to Paris I went, leaving my worries behind for a bit.

It was one of the most memorable work trips I've ever taken. I can't actually tell you anything about what we did for work, but I can tell you that the off-hours sightseeing, the running along the Seine in the early mornings, and the "Allez Les Bleus" chanting during the World Cup finals took my mind away from baby making. Which is why on the last morning of the trip, when I woke up with what I thought was a stomachache, I assumed something I ate the night before at dinner didn't agree with me.

A few minutes later, half-awake on the toilet, I wiped and spotted RED on the toilet paper. No Parisian café noir needed; that sight woke me up faster than any shot of espresso ever could. HOLY SHIT, I have my period. All by myself, no drugs, no curling iron, just me and my ovaries. I danced around my hotel room in celebration, but then mid-jump, I froze.

Never in a million years did I think I'd get my period. I had no feminine products packed with me, no sanitary napkins, no tampons, nothing. After a quick sweep of the hotel bathroom, neither did the hotel. My mood quickly went from New Year's Eve ball-dropping celebratory fun to straight panic.

I sent a message to one of the only other premenopausal females on the trip with me, praying like hell she either had her period right now or was the daughter of a Boy Scout and was always prepared for anything. Thankfully, the latter was true. She had ONE tampon on her, which she graciously offered me.

Grateful for the bailout, that was all I needed to get me through the morning meeting. I'd go to the pharmacy up the street on our lunch break and stock up on tampons. I had already been there earlier in the week with a coworker who needed some allergy medicine, and the woman behind the counter was helpful and spoke English. I'd be good to go before heading to our next stop, Dubai.

Lunchtime rolled around, and I made a beeline for the pharmacy. I walked in and was disappointed to see a man working instead of the woman from the other day. I decided to first peruse by myself to see if I could find what I wanted without having to ask for help. The pharmacies in France are not like your local Walgreens in terms of size. They're more like an oversized walk-in closet, so it doesn't take long to do a full scan of the place. Ultimately, my scan did not turn up any feminine products. Damn it, up to the counter I went.

"Bonjour" was all I had up my sleeve in terms of greeting. It was pretty much all I had up my sleeve in terms of French, so I had to quickly switch to English, asking if he had any feminine products. Well, how lucky was I? This fine man didn't speak a lick of English. I did what any other person speaking to another person who doesn't understand her language. I asked again but this time much louder, as if raising my voice would help him understand my question. Realizing that wasn't getting me anywhere, I started doing hand gestures, drawing a uterus with my fingers across my midsection, and then moving one finger up and down from my belly button to my groin, indicating the flow of blood out of my body. I'm not sure what was more beet red at that point—my period or my cheeks.

Somewhere between outlining the Fallopian tube and miming the traffic flow of the vagina, a woman walked in with her little dog on a leash. Bless her soul, this local spoke English. Taking pity on what I have to imagine looked like a completely hysterical American woman, she offered to help me articulate myself to the pharmacist (not that I really could get much worse).

Once we were all on the same page and he realized what I wanted, HIS face turned beet red, but he quickly shuffled me over to the small shelf near the baby rash creams. (What a logical place for feminine products, I know, how in the world did I miss that?) I picked up a package of tampons that claimed to have thirty-six in there, even though it was practically the size of a deck of playing cards. Eager to get the hell out of Dodge and never see these people again, I paid and ran back to the hotel. I'm pretty sure I paid the equivalent to a bottle of the finest champagne for that box of tampons, but I threw my euros at the man and fled.

Upon opening the package, I found that, yes, indeed there were thirty-six tampons in there, and that's all that was in there. No applicators, just thirty-six actual tampons that looked like little cotton bullets. Manual insertion was the only way to get these babies in there, and I was slowly forgetting why I was so desperate to get my period in the first place. It was starting to become a huge pain in the ass.

I eventually got the hang of those little bullets, and several red-eye flights later, I made it to Dubai and then back home. By the time I got home, one week after Paris, Aunt Flow was gone, and it was time to start charting my cycle and making a baby. I was so beyond relieved to have gotten a period, and with a renewed burst of determination I was ready to get pregnant au naturale.

I was pregnant three months later, and I am convinced it only took that long because I miscalculated my cycle the first two months. It turns out, twenty-eight days is the average cycle, and mine was more like thirty-four days. We had sex every other day to ensure optimal sperm yet not miss our window of opportunity, and afterwards I would lay with my legs straight up in the air, hips propped, willing those little sperm to let gravity help them meet up with my egg faster. I'm not convinced this legs-in-the-air guidance on conception is anything more than an urban legend, but the rule follower in me was still large and in charge and clung to that silliness for dear life.

REDEFINING NORMAL

It's ironic that one goes on the pill to avoid getting pregnant, only to come off the pill and discover that one can't get pregnant. I had assumed all my lady parts worked fine. After all, I got a period like clockwork every twenty-eight days while on the pill.

Well, the period you get while on birth control isn't really a period at all. It's sometimes referred to as withdrawal bleeding and is aptly named because it's your uterus's response to the withdrawal of the synthetic hormones it was receiving daily from your birth control pills.[1] You fooled me! Never did I think I wouldn't be able to get a period after going off birth control since I thought I was experiencing one every month when I was on it!

And, this whole PCOS thing? Apparently, I wasn't alone. According to the CDC, 6%–12% of women have PCOS, making it one of the most common causes of female infertility.[2] Ironically though, it's often misdiagnosed, or perhaps I should say over-diagnosed.[3]

In fact, according to PCOS expert Clare Goodwin, about 25% of women have these cysts on their ovaries, but only 10% actually have PCOS.[4] When I dug into what exactly PCOS was all about, I learned that not only is it sometimes misdiagnosed, but it's also misnamed. The name implies that there are many (poly) cysts on one's ovaries. Well, a "cyst" isn't really the right terminology for what's going on down there. "Cyst-like" would be more appropriate because they are actually eggs that didn't mature enough to be ovulated and they were basically abandoned, and one's ovaries move on to the next potential egg.[5] Okay cool, so the name is misleading, and I'm not even sure I actually had the syndrome?

I didn't stumble upon Clare's work until I was researching for this book well after I had conceived. Her findings, though, validated my rebellion, confirming that conventional medicine jumps straight to drugs and surgery when holistic lifestyle treatments may actually do the same job, if not better, with no risk. She recommends getting your diet, stress, exercise, and sleep under control before turning to drugs such as Clomid.[6]

Sometimes you need to follow a program and put a plan together to achieve an outcome. Other times, you need to rebel against the structure, travel the world, take your mind off things, roll the dice (or spin the Roulette wheel in my case), and trust your body to do what it was made to do. What's important is that we acknowledge infertility is a real problem these days, and there is so much help and support available for couples having trouble conceiving on their own. That being said, if you're uncomfortable or feeling cornered into something, rebel. Turn, get out, and run. Listen to me—this is your life, your body, your future. You do not need do anything that doesn't feel right to you. You're allowed to take some time to yourself to think through things. Remove the pressure; take the batteries out of your biological clock for a bit.

WHAT WORKED FOR ME

There's a good possibility that the timing of when we got pregnant was less about my miscalculation and more about my relaxed mood that month. I mean seriously, how many stories have you heard of people you know who stopped actively trying and then magically became pregnant shortly thereafter? I know many couples whom this happened to, and here I was, cliché as it sounds. Even more cliché, Jack was conceived in Las Vegas while we were on vacation visiting my sister. There was little stress and a whole lot of fun. You could say we defied the whole "what happens in Vegas, stays in Vegas" thing because we sure did bring that fetus home with us!

Secret Weapons

We're going to fast-forward forty weeks in a minute, but before we do, let me summarize my pregnancy with four secret weapons. In my humble opinion, these items were just as important as my prenatal vitamin.

Pregnancy Body Pillow

A hidden secret not shared with you until it's too late and there's no turning back is that when you're pregnant, you're not allowed to sleep on your back, right side, and well, do I even have to tell you that sleeping on your stomach isn't an option? This leaves only your left side, and the further along you are, it starts to get uncomfortable and awkward. Enter, the pregnancy pillow. This giant caterpillar friend is a LIFESAVER, and you will sleep so much better. It'll curl around your back and between your legs, making you feel uber-supported and cozy. Even though you're exhausted all of the time, sleeping is not as easy as you would think!

Immunity Boosters

Another hidden secret is that when you are pregnant, your immune system is shot to shit.7 It's just the beginning of a lifetime of putting your child's needs first and neglecting your own. Getting sick while pregnant is basically inevitable, and you need all the help you can get to keep your immunity up. I had a superfood smoothie every day with a nutrient-dense protein powder, frozen fruit, and almond milk; and I prioritized plenty of sleep (thanks to the pillow). Pre-pregnancy, I did these things as well and I was never sick, like ever. Around my seventh month of pregnancy (after having survived a pretty nasty bout of the common cold) I was delighted to find I had double pink eye.

Annie's Boxed Vegan Mac and Cheese

Pregnancy cravings are a real thing, and I would rather pluck my pubic hairs one by one than actually consume the Yellow 5 and Yellow 6 in Kraft mac and cheese. Give in to your cravings, yet do it in the least harmful way possible to you and your baby. Ironically my cravings were almost always savory and rarely sweet, even though I usually have a total sweet tooth. (I could live on chocolate and chocolate alone.) In case sweet cravings are where you find yourself, I recommend plenty of satisfying yet clean sweet treats! Check out Chocolate Covered Katie's blog, and don't poo-poo the black bean brownies until you've tried them! If you're too tired to prep, grab some Sweet Loren's break and bake fudge brownie cookies. You can even eat the dough right out of the fridge!

Pregnancy Spanx

This has nothing to do with feeling slim, because girlfriend, you won't feel slim a single day of pregnancy. It has everything to do with feeling secure. As that belly grows, you're going to start to worry that it's just going to fall out of you or off you, and it's an unnerving sensation. A pair of pregnancy Spanx do just the trick in keeping everything right where it should be. These are more of a psychological survival item than physical, but I'm all about staying sane.

I'll admit I loved being pregnant. Most of the beginning of my pregnancy was a mix between being proud that we got pregnant (Take THAT, PCOS!) and being paranoid that something bad would happen (oh, and being nauseated at the thought of most foods, except Annie's). I was excited to be a mom and start a family with Justin, and I was ready to embrace all nine (really more like ten, but who's counting) months of pregnancy and tried to treat every day like the gift that it was.

2

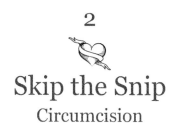

Skip the Snip
Circumcision

ROAD TO REBELLION

I was convinced I was having a girl from early on in my pregnancy, with nothing to back up that conviction other than a bunch of silly old wives' tales' symptoms I was experiencing. I am not one of those women who wants to wait until the big day to find out the sex of her baby, and thankfully Justin wasn't in favor of that option either. I am actually in total awe of those women. I genuinely cannot understand how that if there is information available to be known, to not immediately know it. While I cannot comprehend that type of laid-back approach, I do admire it. However, I wish that when you took a pregnancy test, it didn't just tell you whether you were pregnant, but also included the sex, birthdate, and college GPA of your unborn baby.

Therefore, it should come as no surprise that I signed up for a genetic test, in which around week eleven of pregnancy you have blood work done that checks for chromosome disorders and also determines the baby's sex based on the presence (or lack thereof) of the male chromosome. In case you're reading this and you're early on in your pregnancy, you should know now that you will have blood drawn often. If you start your pregnancy journey skeeved by or queasy at the thought of having blood drawn, you won't even bat an eye by the end of your pregnancy.

At any rate, we received the test results a few days before our annual pre-Christmas trip to the mountains. We agreed we'd wait until we were on vacation to open the envelope and reveal our baby's sex. That plan sounded good until we actually had the envelope from the doctor in hand, and then we couldn't wait any longer. The day before we were leaving, I called Justin on my way home from work, and he asked if I wanted to open it that night. He further proposed that we let the results dictate what we did for dinner that night. If it's a boy, we'd go out to dinner because he'd want to do that like his daddy. If it's a girl, we'd stay in for dinner because she'd want to do that like her mommy. I was totally cool with this proposal because, like I said, I was so sure there was a teeny tiny baby girl in my uterus and I was in no mood to go out to dinner (or eat, or look at food, or even think about food). This was a win-win for Mommy for sure.

When I got home, we sat in front of the Christmas tree and ripped open the envelope. There, right before our eyes, was text that was circled "Y chromosome detected" and right next to it in the doctor's handwriting "It's a boy!" (Probably because 99% of their patients forget what they learned in high school biology and need someone to spell out X versus Y chromosome.) Justin was ecstatic, and I was totally shocked. My mind started reeling. I needed to learn all things boy: sports, trucks, and penises.

It wasn't that day, in fact it wasn't for a few weeks after the big reveal, that the concept of circumcision even crossed my mind. It was a roughly fleeting thought, of which I casually mentioned to Justin, "We'll circumcise the baby, right?" And he said, "Yeah, I guess."

Shortly after that in-depth decision-making session with Justin, I had lunch with a girlfriend who is a role model mama in my eyes. We have many of the same viewpoints and I've talked with her often about pregnancy, birth, etc. We were chit chatting over our meals, and then she nervously asked me about circumcision. She and her husband chose to not circumcise their boys, even though her husband is circumcised. I answered honestly and said that I hadn't given it much thought but that I assumed we would. She told me she had assumed the same, until she started doing a little research into the procedure itself and the rationale (or maybe better stated, "justification") behind it. She was horrified, and once she shared her findings with her husband, he was too. Because she knew I was open minded, she wanted to share her thoughts with me so Justin and I could make a more educated decision. She was nervous bringing it up because she didn't want to seem pushy or judgmental, but I'm incredibly grateful she did.

I went home and told Justin about my lunch conversation, and we decided to watch a documentary on it. Isn't that how most people do research these days? Now, let's take what we learned from this documentary with a grain of salt. There were some STRONG opinions on both sides of the debate, all of which felt a little extreme and a little dramatic to me. I guess that's the cinema business for you—drama sells. However, there were a couple of things I gleaned from the film:

- First, the procedure itself was HORRIFYING. Like, really, really horrifying, even when done as humanely as possible.

> It involved the baby being strapped down, skin being separated that was described as a fingernail being removed from a finger, and then a ten-day recovery period where every time the baby urinates, it burns.[1]

- Second, no one could provide a solid medical reason why it needed to be done. The abstract, limited studies weren't convincing me that bullet one above was worth it. The weak arguments against hygiene, UTIs, penile cancer, and HIV weren't swaying me.

Redefining Normal

My curiosity was piqued, and I set out to understand the origination of what was quickly becoming the most disturbing procedure I'd ever heard of.

Lo and behold, I uncovered some pretty interesting history of circumcision, which seemed to go back to the beginning of time. In fact, the practice is so old, it's hard to pinpoint its origin, although many of the earliest accounts point to the Egyptians.[2] Exact origination was irrelevant for me, the fact being it's been in practice for a long, long time and everyone knows old habits die hard. What was common among all accounts was that circumcision was done to young men originally around the time they hit adolescence, or perhaps more accurately, puberty. It was viewed as a sacrifice, an opportunity to show their manliness by sucking it up and taking it, trying not to show any signs of pain, often with the intent to control their sex drive.[3] (It's hard to imagine that last part is really effective.)

Some direct quotes on the ritual origination include:

- "...served most of the spiritual purposes of castration without depriving a man of his fertility."[4]

- "...primarily to control masturbation in adolescents and young boys."[5]

Then, as we evolved to modern medicine:

- "There was a strong dogmatic belief that it was necessary to prevent penile cancer."[6]

- "...offers protection against sexually transmitted diseases..."[7]

However, all I could hear was the ghost of Hippocrates whispering to me, "First, do no harm."

Today, it is one of the most common medical surgeries in the United States, although the percentage of male infants who are circumcised is declining.[8] The current American Academy of Pediatrics statement on circumcision explains: "Although health benefits are not great enough to recommend routine circumcision for all male newborns, the benefits of circumcision are sufficient to justify access to this procedure for families choosing it and to warrant third-party payment for circumcision of male newborns." This latest statement, dated 2012, is an update to the 1999 statement, which did not include the piece about access and payment.[9]

The current statement also reads: "Parents ultimately should decide whether circumcision is in the best interests of their male child. They will need to weigh medical information in the context of their own religious, ethical, and cultural beliefs and practices".[10] While I agree with the concept that parents should ultimately make the decision, I think it's a little unfair that they are not receiving any guidance from medical experts and that they are left to "weigh medical information" without a medical degree.

As mentioned, the 2012 statement is an update from the 1999 statement, which more clearly stated that the benefits don't outweigh the risks.[11] This 1999 viewpoint is more in line with many other countries' current day viewpoints. In fact, there are several countries that don't take an impartial approach and actually advise against it, including Holland, Germany, Austria, Switzerland[12], and Canada.[13] So, why is it that we're all on the same planet, with access to the same medical information, and birthing the same species (the last time I checked anyway), yet getting conflicting advice on how to treat our newborn sons?

At its core, the procedure can be summed up as follows. First, the foreskin is separated from the head of the penis.[14] You may be surprised to hear this part; perhaps you assumed the foreskin was always retractable, but that is not true. When a baby boy is born, the foreskin is basically sealed to the penis, with just a small hole opening for urination. It doesn't naturally separate, giving it the ability to retract, until later in life.[15]

Next, once the foreskin is separated, a straight line is cut down the shaft toward the body, and finally at the base, a circle is cut around the shaft to remove it entirely. The amount that is removed varies by baby and by the person performing the procedure, but it is often surprising how much skin is removed.

Did I mention that the entire time the baby is restrained, either strapped down in a contraption or held still by another person? A local anesthetic is typically used to numb the penis, either a topical or an injection.[16]

I was swayed even more when I found out that circumcision often has an impact on breastfeeding. This is because, while even if numbed, the procedure can be both painful and scary for your baby. Naturally, newborns who undergo painful surgical procedures have high levels of stress hormones which speed up their heart rates and suppress the high oxytocin levels that would trigger their innate impulses to nurse.[17] Although I don't see how this is really unique to newborns, I'm pretty sure stress is a general human reaction to pain. Regardless, I didn't like the idea it could impact breastfeeding, something I was adamant on doing.

Then, there is the whole at-home treatment afterward. This is what was in my generic take-home pamphlet from the hospital on the post-op care: "Baby's penis will be swollen and dark red in color. Within 24 hours, the penis will be covered with a crusty discharge for about 7 days." Friends, can we talk about what a shitstorm it is the first couple of weeks at home with a newborn? As a mama, if you had a vaginal birth, you're wearing adult diapers and bleeding like a stuffed pig. If you had a C-section, you're tending to a huge incision AND also wearing adult diapers (the bleeding doesn't discriminate between vaginal and C-section births). If you're nursing, you are also dealing with leaky, swollen boobs, and if you're extra lucky, cracked nipples. I wasn't feeling like we needed to add taking care of a swollen, crusty, discharging, tiny penis into the mix.

Even the pamphlet assumes most parents will circumcise, as the real estate on the page given to education on a circumcised penis versus education on an uncircumcised penis is more than double. It felt like a subtle, subliminal message implying not circumcising is the road less traveled.

Just when I thought I couldn't be horrified any further, I concluded that the root of all evil, money, is a motive behind the medical industry pushing circumcision in the United States. Hence, this further supports the higher number of circumcisions performed in the U.S. versus the rest of the world. For one, it's a procedure that the medical industry can charge for, and because it's covered by insurance, the bill is guaranteed to be paid.[18] And two, the foreskin is sold to beauty lines to be used in products such as anti-aging face creams.[19]

Yes, go ahead and reread that paragraph. Am I in the twilight zone? You mean to tell me we routinely cut off the tips of newborns' penises, convince ourselves the procedure doesn't hurt them (physically nor psychologically), charge the parents and ultimately their insurance companies, and then package up the skin to send to skincare manufacturers and various other research centers? Are we THAT disillusioned as a society?

As a last-ditch effort, in case folks can't get behind the need to reduce masturbation, UTIs, and penile cancer, hygiene is thrown in as a rationale for circumcising—implying if we don't do it, the baby won't be clean or be as easy to clean.[20] News flash: Has anyone looked at a vagina lately? There are more nooks, crannies, and flaps in there that need to be cleaned but you don't see anyone chopping that up. (Side note: female circumcision is a real thing and was just as horrifying for me to read about. I'm not going to go into it in detail here, but there are some cultures who do practice circumcision on women, as well.)[21]

WHAT WORKED FOR ME

No matter how you slice it (definitely no pun intended), and believe me the information out there will spin it every which way, we're essentially talking elective surgery. It's adding unnecessary trauma on top of an already eventful time for a newborn. (Can you even imagine what traveling down the birth canal is like?) Absolutely, there are ways to conduct the procedure to cause as little pain as possible to the baby, including a numbing cream or local anesthetic. There are also plenty of ways to conduct the procedure that do little to eliminate the pain. I've read many accounts where even if a local anesthetic was used, oftentimes it wasn't completely numbing, or in some cases sufficient time was not permitted to allow the local anesthetic to take full effect.

I asked myself, if this isn't truly required, why am I subjecting my brand-new baby to numbing chemicals? Don't I have enough to worry about, like latching and sleeping (more on those topics later)?

Is your head spinning? Mine was. Look, I'm not judging (remember this is a judgement-free zone) if you have some personal or religious belief that is driving you to do this. The thing is, I didn't. I had no reason to do so, and after all I had uncovered, everything inside me was yelling to not do it.

I was a big fan of my nurse practitioner, so during one of my routine prenatal visits I asked her about it. She paused and answered relatively objectively with the same bullshit I had found in my research regarding the limited pros and cons (including social norms) and that ultimately, it's our preferential decision. My husband, ever the crowdsourcer, followed up with, "What do you see most people do?" I'm normally not a fan of this question, but I'm so glad he asked it. Her response was, "Majority of deliveries I've done, the parents have their babies circumcised. Except for the three years I lived abroad. I only did one circumcision, and it was for a mother who was vacationing from the States and unexpectedly had her baby while traveling." My friends, I rest my case.

I read that "...circumcision in America is a cultural practice, chosen by parents for social conformity or aesthetics."[22] I was starting to believe that to be true. A rationale in the social norm arena for circumcision is that parents want their baby to look like daddy. Again, I'm a woman so I can't relate, but I don't remember ever comparing vaginas with my mom. Maybe we did and it was unmemorable? As far as boobs go, every girl sees her mom's, sister's, and girlfriends' boobs, and you show me two pairs of boobs that are identical, and I'll give you ten bucks. Needless to say, my experience with this look-alike reasoning was limited, so I asked my husband and my dad. My husband rolled his eyes at me and told me he didn't remember ever having a genital comparing occasion with his father. My dad, never one to turn down the opportunity to tell a story, did distinctly remember seeing his dad's penis for the first time.

My grandpa, born at home in the early 1920s, was not

circumcised. He and my dad were at an outdoor fair when my dad was around seven or eight, and my dad told my grandpa that he had to go to the bathroom. Being manly men, my grandpa found a spot behind a barn where they could take a leak. Out come the penises, and lo and behold, according to my dad, my grandpa's "had a case". My dad, always one to bluntly ask a question, asked, "Why does your penis look like that?" My grandpa, a man of very few words, usually curt and gruff, said, "Your mom had yours cut off when you were a baby so that you would always be clean." That answer worked for my dad, and life moved on.

While my husband didn't have a show-and-tell with his father, he did play Division I hockey (Yes, I married a stud.), and he had countless locker room stories of those who had a "covered wagon" or an "anteater". He often played with Canadians and Europeans, and he said they were rarely circumcised. He said there was no shame in the game in the locker room, meaning anything goes, and they'd all constantly be poking fun at each other. He even went as far as explaining to me what a piss bomb was. I think I would have been fine to have gone through life never knowing about this "trick", but since my eyes have been opened, it's only fair I open your eyes too. The uncircumcised guys would urinate while holding their foreskin shut, so that it all pooled in there, and then release the hold and spray the other guys with their pee. If that's not a reason to keep your baby boy intact, I'm not sure what is.

All joking aside, I asked if the teasing was in good humor or if it was malicious. The mama bear in me didn't want my little boy to be made fun of if he were "different". He said it was always in good humor, and never did he feel like the guys were being bullied, nor did he think any differently of them because they weren't circumcised.

I ultimately told Justin I felt like he should have the final say on this decision (a rarity in our marriage for sure) because at the end of the day the majority of penis topics will be his responsibility to handle. (I have to draw the line somewhere!) Now if you know anything about Justin and me, we're on the opposite ends of the spectrum on decision making. I'm pretty cut and dry; I can easily make a decision and almost rarely have buyer's remorse. Justin, on the other hand, will agonize over every decision, and usually he doesn't do the actually deciding until the eleventh hour. Which is why, on Jack's birthday, the verdict was still unsettled.

3

You Pay for What You Get
Birth Story

ROAD TO REBELLION

As we dive into the day my son came down the birth canal, let's talk a little bit about how I didn't want things to go. (Who named it the birth canal? It's misleading, completely implying that he should have arrived in a Venetian gondola, delivered by one of those adorable Italian men wearing a striped shirt and a bandana bib, while I sat there sipping Prosecco.)

Today's society leads us to believe birth is painful and that there's no way we can do it without some numbing drugs. I have so many girlfriends and have heard so many women tell their birth story and use lines like "I couldn't wait for the drugs" and "They almost wouldn't give me an epidural and I was freaking out". Unfortunately, some of my closest girlfriends have stories that ended in an unwanted C-section or the necessary use of forceps because mama was too exhausted and numbed to push from the effect of the drugs.

For such a large and monumental event in my life, drugs didn't feel like the appropriate course of action. And real talk, the idea of my legs being numb from an epidural freaked me out more than the idea of my vagina dilating ten centimeters.

By the end of my pregnancy, I was ready—mentally and physically—to have this baby naturally and understood all the benefits of a drug-free labor, skin-to-skin contact with your newborn, and early breastfeeding.

So, imagine how I felt at my forty-week, five-day OB-GYN appointment when my favorite nurse practitioner came in the exam room and said to me, "We want you to get induced today." My heart sank, and I could feel the pit of my stomach. It didn't seem real, almost like I was watching a movie or reading one of the many less-than-ideal birth stories. Just three days ago, I had been in for a visit and everything looked fine—my doctor even told me he'd let me go all the way until forty-two weeks before inducing me. I was prepared to wait out the full forty-two weeks and let this baby come when he was good and ready. Plus, earlier that morning, I started having contractions and was timing them throughout the day, so I felt like the baby was starting to prepare for his arrival.

"Why?" I quietly, desperately asked her. She was more than adequately prepared with an answer, or more like a laundry list of reasons:

- My amniotic fluid was lower than they'd like; they want it between 5 and 20 cm, and mine was 4.75 cm.

- My baby was measuring 6 lbs., 11 oz, which put him in the 25th percentile—no cause for alarm by itself, but back at my 32-week appointment, he was measuring in the 60th percentile.

- My blood pressure had been creeping up each visit, and my face (apparently) looked puffy.

- I'm past due.

My internal reaction: gulp. My external reaction: "What if I say I don't want to be induced today?" I mentioned this was my favorite nurse practitioner, but let me elaborate. She has about forty years of experience in this field and was a midwife forever before joining my practice. I always trusted her opinion. She's not one to jump to conventional medicine, and she understands the benefit of letting nature run its course. Her answer to me was all I needed to hear, "I'm pretty liberal, and I'm telling you, you need to do this." She and the doctors were worried that my placenta had stopped doing its job (hence, the low fluid and small-for-gestation baby measurements), and they didn't want to take any chances. They wanted me to go to the hospital and have Cervidil for twelve hours overnight, then start a Pitocin drip in the morning.

I was familiar with Cervidil and Pitocin from my research, and they were two words I never wanted to hear when it was my turn. They were certainly two words I didn't want to hear together in the same sentence. Cervidil is another one of those jump starters—this one ripens your cervix and accelerates dilation. Pitocin is synthetic oxytocin and is given to women to intensify and speed up contractions. Neither one was in my plans for game day.

Okay, I'm getting induced. Here it comes, my worst nightmare. I reunited with Justin who was sitting in the waiting room, and we went up to the receptionist to schedule my induction with the hospital. She told us the hospital was "really busy" but that she'd push to get us in. She was treating it like a business transaction, and I was treating it like a death sentence. Neither of us were appropriate in our treatment of the situation, but nevertheless she got us set up with a 3 p.m. induction that day. She told me I could have no food or drink starting at 1 p.m. until I had the baby. I did the math in my head, realizing that's going to be a long time without water, and last time I checked I wasn't a camel despite my giant hump.

We went out to the car, and it started pouring, which felt appropriate for the current situation. I had a good cry and then pulled myself together, knowing the only way to get through this was to stay positive. I called my mom and told her, and she said she'd meet us at the hospital after work. I didn't tell any other family. For one, I really didn't want to have to talk about it. And two, I didn't want the pressure of people knowing I was sitting in the hospital, waiting for the Cervidil to ripen/open my cervix. Justin and I agreed that in the morning, when they started the Pitocin, we'd tell everyone else that we were at the hospital.

While I didn't have much of an appetite, I knew that I had to eat, and more importantly I knew I had to eat good-for-you food. I was about to start a marathon. Off to Whole Foods we went, where I loaded up a big salad and snagged a granola bar for my 1 p.m. on-the-dot snack. After lunch, Justin and I decided we'd go home and pack a more comprehensive suitcase, now that we knew what we were in for. We grabbed everything, including Yahtzee, playing cards, and Justin's laptop to watch movies. We figured we needed something to help pass the time while the Cervidil did its thing.

Driving to the hospital felt a little strange. I think we both envisioned the hospital ride would be stressful, with me having painful contractions in the front seat. Even when we got to the hospital, it was anticlimactic. We walked up to the Labor and Delivery ward like we were checking in to a hotel.

True to what we heard earlier, they were fully booked. Instead of getting a delivery room, we were put into a small (emphasis on small) exam room that didn't even have a private bathroom. We were ignored for a bit once we got there, but finally our nurse, Allison, came in. She was a sweetheart, but a bit of a train wreck. Overwhelmed by how busy they were, she made a mess inserting my IV—blood everywhere in the room and on me, including in my engagement ring, turning my diamond temporarily pink. I never even got a wristband until much later in the night. My mom arrived around 6 p.m. We tried to send her home, telling her it was going to be a long, uncomfortable, uneventful night, but she wasn't hearing it. So, all three of us settled into this cozy room, waiting for the Cervidil insert.

Finally at 6:30 p.m., Kathy, the resident midwife, came to insert the Cervidil. In case you haven't researched the shit out of induction drugs, allow me to explain. Cervidil is like a tampon made of sandpaper, manually inserted (not unlike like the bullet tampons in Paris), and it stays in your vagina for twelve hours, releasing something that is supposed to ripen your cervix. She told me I may experience some cramping as the evening progressed, and that if I were in too much pain, they had a Benadryl cocktail I could take to ease the pain. She also emphasized that this was not the time to be a hero and turn down the pain medication since I had a long road ahead of me. Great, thanks for the words of encouragement, Kathy.

A few uneventful hours went by, and I continued to monitor my contractions which were coming closer together, but still manageable. At this point, Allison went home for the night, and I met Sarah, my overnight nurse. Sarah, it turned out, was definitely an angel on earth. About one and a half hours into the Cervidil, she told me I could have water and some clear liquid "foods". Hallelujah! Nightmares of not eating until three days later were over! I happily indulged in ice cold water and two apple juices. (What a SPLURGE!) Shortly after that feast, she came into our shoebox of a room and announced she scored us a real Labor and Delivery room, one with actual square footage worth noting, and more than just a folding chair for your entourage. I was ecstatic, mostly for Justin and my mom's sake.

As we transitioned to our new room, things started to heat up for me. I was suddenly overcome by the need to have a bowel movement. So much so that I said to Justin, if I don't get to the bathroom soon, I'm going to shit on this bed. In response, he came over and unplugged my monitors so that I could freely move about and get to our (private!) bathroom. True love. From there things escalated quickly. Those manageable contractions were no longer manageable. They were coming fast and furious and painfully so. Sarah called Kathy in, and Kathy said to me, yes, you could be experiencing some side effect cramping from the Cervidil, but we're monitoring your uterus activity and what you're describing as intense pain is not quite at the level for how we define intense pain. She proceeded to remind me about the Benadryl cocktail and left the room.

My heart sank and my confidence weakened. I always thought I had a high tolerance for pain but maybe I was wrong. (I once broke my ankle and hobbled around for three days before finally going to urgent care, only to find out it was broken and needed surgery). Justin was starting to worry that I was having a bad reaction to the Cervidil based on what his Google search produced, and he and my mom convinced me I should take the pain medication. (Note to self: Never, ever let your husband have access to the internet in the Labor and Delivery room.) I caved and said okay. I was in immense pain; I felt like a giant hand was wrapped around my midsection in a vice grip, only letting up for a few seconds before tightening the hold tenfold, and I was nervous about how much more work I had in front of me.

Sarah and Kathy came back in to give me the cocktail, which was really just a pill to swallow. I asked Kathy how long until I felt some relief, and she told me about thirty minutes. I watched the clock like a hawk, in between my ninety-second long, one-minute apart contractions. At this point I had to hang on to my mom's neck or Justin's neck in a half-hug, and talking through the contractions was no longer an option. Thirty minutes went by, then forty-five minutes, and finally I said to Sarah, "I don't feel any better. In fact, I feel much worse." She asked me if she could put her hands where I was having pain, and I said of course. She held my lower abdomen through one of my contractions, and then she said, "Let me get Kathy. That is really strong." Sarah, my angel.

A few minutes later (I think? Time sort of stood still and flew all at the same time.), Kathy and Sarah returned. Kathy said to me, "We're going to take out the Cervidil. You're in way too much pain, and it's not supposed to be that bad on the drug." Then, way more flippant than I would have liked, "Oh, and since your cramping is in your lower abdomen, we're not picking it up on the monitor (which was placed around my upper abdomen), and Sarah let me know just how intense it was." Moment of triumph for me. My tolerance for pain WAS really good. However, quite honestly, I was in too much pain to gloat. I just wanted anything to relieve me.

At this point it was 12:30 a.m. The Cervidil had been in me for six hours. We were all hopeful I was well-dilated at this point, and maybe that's why I was in so much pain. Kathy took out the Cervidil and checked me—barely two centimeters. Completely deflating. Again I asked her, "How long until I feel some relief?" She said thirty, maybe forty-five minutes. She told me she wanted me to rest once I felt relief so that I was in better shape for when they started the Pitocin in the morning. Again I watched the clock, but relief never came. In fact, it got worse. My contractions were on top of each other, no down time in between. I was panicked that there was no way I was going to make it through the night, much less through an entire day of Pitocin and labor the following day. I asked Sarah if there was anything else they could do. She told me there was one other drug they could put through my IV that slows down contractions. (They give it to women who are going into preterm labor.) I said I'd take it. My drug-free labor was slowly fading from view, but I was also trying to keep myself afloat.

The drug, thank goodness, actually worked. My contractions expanded to about ten minutes apart, and in between I would fade into "sleep", wake up, manage through the contraction, and fade back out. That lasted about one hour. Then we were right back to where we were before, and then some. Like a broken record, I asked if there was anything else they could do. Unfortunately, my only other option was an epidural. I said absolutely not, not this early. I didn't want to be immobile, have a catheter, etc. I said no way. Instead, I asked if I could go into the tub.

Sarah told me I could, but that the jets weren't working. Bless her heart. I said to her "Sarah, I'm not looking for a day spa experience, just a little bit of relief." I had read about the benefits of being in water, and my OB-GYN had recommended it as well. So splish splash I went. Justin came into the bathroom with me, sitting outside the tub and holding me as I draped my body over the side. The tub itself actually did help. What didn't help was the woman in the room next to mine, screaming so loud I could hear her through the wall. Still to this day I never confirmed if she was giving birth or being stabbed to death with a machete. Regardless, it was difficult to Zen out with that as my white noise.

I spent about forty-five minutes in the tub, trying hard to practice the hypnobirthing techniques I had spent weeks reading about. I was doing pretty well (all things considered), and Justin was excellent encouragement. Then I suddenly felt like I had to throw up, and with each contraction I found myself needing to kneel upright, almost as if something was going to come out of me, like I was going to shit out of my vagina. I had this split-second moment where I thought, they say if you throw up or feel like you're going to throw up, you are probably in transition. Transition is the final stage of dilation when a woman moves to fully dilated. Could it be? I quickly dismissed the thought. There was no way. I was only two centimeters a few hours ago. At the same time, Sarah came in and said that they had to monitor me; I had been in the tub for a while not hooked up to the monitors. I was needing a change of scenery (more like sound-ery) anyway. I got out of the tub and peed in the toilet. While seated, Sarah felt my contractions again with her hand. She said she was going to have Kathy check my dilation.

We went back to the bed and waited for Kathy. My mom was asleep in the guest recliner, snoring. God bless her. At least someone was getting a few minutes of shut-eye. Kathy came in, checked me, and proclaimed, "Oh wow, you're nine centimeters dilated!" My mom popped up from her slumber like a jack-in-the-box and shouted, "Nine centimeters?!" Justin teared up, and I silently applauded myself. I freaking did it. That whole time I was in active labor without knowing it, and now we were here. It was go time.

Kathy then asked me if I wanted an epidural. I didn't respond right away. I was trying to digest the fact that I made it through dilation and transition without even knowing it, and I could now see the finish line. She was babbling about the pros and cons of an epidural, and I mumbled, "I don't want one." She didn't hear me and kept talking, so I said louder, "I don't want one." She looked surprised, considering I was acting like death was upon me earlier in the evening (morning?). She said, "Okay then, let's call the doctor. By the way, you're really more like ten centimeters dilated. I just didn't want you to freak out if you did want an epidural." (Kathy was really batting a thousand.)

Just like that, we went from not a whole lot going on to the room feeling like Grand Central Station. You could feel all the energy and anticipation in the room. Sarah told me to get into whatever position I was comfortable in, and when the urge to push came, push. I was pleasantly surprised. I didn't realize my hospital was supportive of "unassisted pushing". Brownie points for them. It almost made up for the jets not working on the tub (kidding). Meanwhile, Sarah was off in the corner clanking and banging and preparing something, but I was too focused to pay her much mind.

The position I was most comfortable in was half-kneeling, half table top. She was right. The urge to push completely takes over and there's no stopping it. At some point my on-call OB-GYN, Dr. C., came into the room. I know the time was roughly around 5:30 a.m. They told me I had to lie back down for a minute for Dr. C. to check me. I complied, and quickly Dr. C. said, "Oh yeah, I'll go scrub in." That was a great sign for me. It meant she knew this baby was going to come on her shift, which was over at 7 a.m.!

I went back into my comfortable position, but suddenly everyone was noticing that was not comfortable for the baby. Everyone but me anyway. Thankfully, I was oblivious to the baby monitoring. I kept hearing, "The baby doesn't like that position," and each time I heard it, there was more and more concern in their voices. "Okay, well what position does the baby like because I'll hang from the ceiling if that's what it'll take!" I thought.

Shortly after, Dr. C. announced, "Okay I'm sorry, Laura, but we have to do this the old-fashioned way. The stirrups are coming out, and you're going to have to push. We need to get this baby out ASAP." My reaction was twofold:

1. I wasn't upset by that news because I had assumed that was how they were going to make me deliver anyway, the unassisted pushing was a pleasant surprise.

2. Shit, something is wrong with the baby.

I immediately did whatever they told me. Into the stirrups my feet went, with Sarah holding my left leg and Justin holding my right. Dr. C. told me she was going to give me a perineal massage and that it might hurt a bit. I told her we were way past the point of caring about pain. Next, she told me I had to push when I felt a contraction: breathe in, hold your breath, and push three times. Then she said, "Push like you're taking a poop." So, during my next contraction I breathed in and tried to push like I was pooping, except I don't poop in this position. I was having the hardest time making the mind-body connection, and my pushing was horrible. I could tell she was not only disappointed but concerned that if that was all I had in me, this wasn't going to work.

I tried to gain composure, reminded myself that this baby's life depends on me, and I gave it a go a second time. This time I nailed it; I could tell by her encouragement. Once I had it, I went full force. I pushed so hard that after a few contractions, Dr. C. casually told Sarah to give me some oxygen through the face mask in between contractions to prevent me from hyperventilating.

Justin was cheering me on like it was a sporting event. His was one of the only voices in the room I homed in on. After less than thirty minutes of pushing, out emerged my precious boy...with the umbilical cord wrapped not once, but twice, around his neck. There was no ceremonial cutting of the cord by Justin. Dr. C. snipped it immediately to free him and passed him to the NICU nurses, who were waiting right in the same room as me, next to my bed, unbeknownst to me. Everyone held their breath while the NICU nurses worked to give Jack his first breath.

I laid there surprisingly calm, trying not to panic. Dr. C. also seemed calm, so I told myself everything had to be all right. I felt in my gut things were going to be okay. Seconds later (I found out later it was twenty-eight seconds, to be exact), I heard Jack cry for the first time, and my heart swelled. He was okay! Once they were comfortable with how he was breathing, he was placed on my chest for our first look. I felt joy in finally seeing each other after being one for so many months. All the horrible, scary, overwhelming, and uncomfortable moments from the previous twelve hours quickly faded into the background as I soaked in this tiny wonder.

He was incredibly alert considering the disruption to his previously dull existence. Albeit he was the first baby I saw in the flesh directly after birth, so I have nothing to compare it to. He cranked his neck up to better see me, trying to figure out what in the world was going on. His little cry sounded like a pterodactyl, and his fingers were as wrinkled as a ninety-year-old woman. And, his hair! My word, it was strawberry blond even though both of his parents are brunettes (one could argue my husband's hair is black). This is the first of Jack's many traits that scream, "I'm a unique little sparkler!" Naturally, I thought he was the most perfect thing I'd ever seen.

Friends, I was elated. It's the only way to describe the feeling I had after pulling an all-nighter, not eating anything for a ridiculously long period of time for someone who normally snacks around the clock, and meeting my first-born beautiful baby boy. I can personally attest to what they say about postpartum hormones making you feel like you're able to flap your arms and fly when you have a natural birth. When I tell you that nothing was going to bring me down, I mean it. However, there was one thing that I would have lost my shit on the nurses for had I not been the world's happiest woman at that moment.

As they were cleaning me, I asked one of the nurses if I could have the IV taken out of my hand, since we never ended up needing to administer any drugs or fluids. She casually says to me, "Oh, we started a Pitocin drip after you delivered to help contract your uterus." I was dumbfounded. While, yes, it had been a whirlwind, I don't ever remember anyone asking nor telling me about this. I'm sure in one of the forty forms I signed upon arrival I gave consent, but I was furious (as furious as the happiest woman on the planet can be). I didn't say anything in the moment, but I took note to bitch about this at a later date to my husband.

As we transitioned from the labor and delivery room to the postpartum room, it became apparent that I was the talk of the staff break lounge. It was one of those times where those around you are making you feel like a super star, even though you don't feel like you did anything monumental. Yet every time someone new would come in to see me or check on the baby, they'd say things like, "Oh, you're the one who had the baby in less than twelve hours!" or "You're the one who pushed for less than thirty minutes," or my favorite one which was every time my nurse came in to check my stomach, she'd comment, "I can't believe how much your stomach has flattened out already." Alison, my little scatterbrained IV inserter, came back on shift at 7 a.m. and came running into my room proclaiming, "I can't believe you did it so fast!" What did I do that was so abnormal?

REDEFINING NORMAL

It would make my day if you carved out eighty-seven minutes of your life to watch the documentary The Business of Being Born. It's a 2008 documentary, so while a bit outdated, it was the catalyst to all my research on induced births and was one of the main reasons why I was so hell-bent on having a natural birth.

I went back through my reading log and noted over twenty books I had read on the topic of natural birthing. That's just books; it doesn't count the podcasts, journal articles, and countless anecdotes I received from solicited (and many unsolicited) stories from friends and acquaintances. (Can we sidebar for a minute and talk about how there are so many women out there who, upon interacting with a pregnant woman, get the worst case of verbal diarrhea and want to tell them EVERY bad thing that happened to them during pregnancy and the early days of motherhood? Listen, love, I'm not your diary nor your therapist. Please save that story for someone who isn't about to be a first-time mom.) I digress.

Hypnobirthing, invented by one of the OG rebel mamas, Marie Mongan[1], takes the cake as probably the coolest concept I read about natural childbirth. Mongan was inspired by Grantly Dick-

Read's theory of eliminating the fear-tension-pain syndrome (a man before his time, author of legendary *Childbirth Without Fear*). Mongan created a spin on hypnotherapy, coined it hypnobirthing, and has helped thousands of women each year align with their own innate capacity to give birth. Hypnobirthing techniques teach women to release fear and practice affirmations and visualization for a peaceful, natural birth.[2]

Intrigued by my short stint in the bathtub? Laboring in water kept coming up again and again as I was reading about birth. Warm water is comforting in general, and when a woman labors in the tub, she's relieved from gravity's pull.[3] The result? Her body is much calmer, and instead of releasing stress-related hormones (which can slow down labor), her body will produce endorphins instead. (Yup, you guessed it, these will help move labor along.)[4]

I also highly recommend anything that Ina May Gaskin has written. In addition to her books, she has a TED Talk and she's been honored with many awards for being the most legendary midwife to ever walk the face of the earth. She even has an obstetric procedure named for her, the Gaskin Maneuver, to help when baby's head is out but the shoulders are stuck.[5] I would literally do anything to go back in time and be able to birth at the farm under her care. Warning: all things Ina May are SUPER hippy, which I understand can turn some of you off, but fight through it. She started in the 1970s (delivering babies in a school bus!)[6], so what do you expect? Peace, love, and babies.

I wasn't just being a hormonal witch when I was miffed about the Pitocin drip. One of the reasons I wanted to avoid Pitocin was because the synthetic drug does not give you that beautiful high I told you about earlier, which you now know does wonders for both you and baby, and it also reduces your natural oxytocin temporarily.[7]

I'd be doing you a disservice if I didn't dive into the C-section craze in the United States. I recognize it's not common for women to have a scheduled C-section as part of their birth plan, yet the U.S. cesarean rate has increased substantially over the past few decades. According to the CDC, almost 32% of babies were delivered by cesarean in 2019[8], an increase from about 21% in 1996.[9] Over half of the increase is among first-time moms, and most of these C-sections are done for more subjective reasons such as slow progress in labor.[10]

An interesting find was that the World Health Organization (WHO) has stated, "Cesarean rates need not be more than 10–15% of all births. When medically necessary, a cesarean section can effectively prevent maternal and newborn mortality. Two studies show that when caesarean section rates rise towards 10% across a population, the number of maternal and newborn deaths decreases. When the rate goes above 10%, there is no evidence that mortality rates improve."[11] Then why are about one-third of births in the U.S. C-sections?

There are all sorts of theories debated. Some say doctors are tempted by the convenience of a C-section. After all, it's much easier for planning purposes to know exactly when a baby will be born and how long it will take to be born.[12] There is also a correlation between an increase in high-risk pregnancies and an increase in C-sections.[13] This begs the question, is our decline in overall health partially to blame? (Eat your veggies, ladies!) Others think it's a conspiracy by medical professionals because a cesarean brings in more revenue than a vaginal birth.[14] Regardless of the reason, it's become too common of a practice that women think it's normal or actually an option (scheduling it like it's a hair appointment) when the complications and aftermath can be incredibly challenging for mamas during an already challenging time.

In Jennifer Margulis's eye-opening book The Business of Baby, she reveals, "The United States spends more money on health care than any other country in the world. Hospital charges related to pregnancy, delivery, and infant care are among the top five most expensive conditions requiring hospitalization. Pregnancy-related hospital costs are second only to coronary heart disease."[15] I wish I could say that wasn't the case for me, but my hospital bills were nothing short of shocking.

WHAT WORKED FOR ME

I was perplexed by why everyone in the hospital was so blown away by my fast labor, and it didn't dawn on me until later. Sure, I like to think of myself as a rock star, but I really didn't do anything spectacular except let nature run its course. When you don't intervene unnecessarily (To all my C-section mamas who were in life-or-death moments, that is what I consider necessary intervention.), your body takes over and does all the work for you. (Remember prolactin and oxytocin—they were big helpers). It's your mind that needs the support; it will either help or hurt you, so I strongly encourage some type of mental prep beforehand (like hypnobirthing) to prevent yourself from scaring the bejesus out of you.

I was in a hospital that touted themselves multiple times during my hospital tour as being supportive of natural birthing methods, yet drugs were still pushed on me far too often and quickly. These nurses aren't evil (Well, the jury is still out on Kathy, who by the way, I was hugging before I left the delivery room - that's how caught up in the moment I was), it's just the way they're trained, and quite frankly it's still the offerings that most mamas want to hear. I am totally supportive of all my mamas out there who need a little something-something to mask the pain IF they understand both the pros and the cons beforehand. An informed decision is a respected decision in my eyes. If we allow ourselves to just follow the herd, or worse feel pressured into a decision, only later to find ourselves with regret or complications, then we're doing ourselves a disservice.

Speaking of decision, Jack was BORN, and we were still telling the nurses, "We're not sure," when asked, what felt like repeatedly, if we were circumcising him. In fact, the question was often posed more like, "You're circumcising him, right? It doesn't say one way or another on his chart here," as if there were only one right answer.

Finally, we were at the point where putting off our answer was no longer an option, and when asked the last time if we were circumcising Jack, Justin simply answered with "no". My heart swelled, and I'm pretty sure I let out a big sigh of relief. You might find this hard to believe, but I didn't pressure, bully, or influence him. I truly wanted him to be okay with where he landed, and I remained neutral and accepting while he thought through it (maybe another rare moment in our marriage, if I'm being honest).

I asked him what helped him with the decision, and he said, "I couldn't handle the thought of someone unnecessarily taking a can opener to my son's manhood."

Such a way with words, I know, but I couldn't agree more with him. The verdict was in. We had concluded that for us, it felt like a hoax and unnecessary, and we rebelled. My baby has all the skin he was born with, and I dodged a big dose of mom guilt. (Why didn't anyone warn me how real the mom guilt is?! More on that later.)

Many months later, when researching for this book, I came across a quote from Dr. Spock, aka Mr. Baby for mamas of generations past when they were in the throes of parenthood, who originally recommended circumcision in some of his early work. But as time passed and myths were debunked and research proved no real benefits, he was quoted in a 1989 article in *Redbook* magazine saying, "My own preference, if I had the good fortune to have another son, would be to leave his little penis alone."[16] It's almost as eloquent as my husband's can opener analogy.

Something that has helped me often: Instinct versus instruction. Rarely will our instinct betray us. Instruction, on the other hand, often assumes a one-size-fits-all, which is not even close to the case when it comes to your birth story (and definitely not the case when it comes to your baby, either).

Another reflection point is how so many of these medical

professionals deliver news so matter-of-factly. It feels transactional, and while I know I was just one of many patients they spoke to in a day, this was a huge deal in my life.

Here I am preaching to trust our bodies and trust our gut instincts, and even I needed that reminder when caught up in the moment. I wish that stupid computer could have slapped Kathy in the face—technology is wonderful when we use it correctly. As prepared as I was, it was such a humbling experience to realize there are so many different ways situations could go, that I was naïve to think I could be prescriptive in my birth plan. You should rather have a birth ideal, but not a rigid plan. Be open to several options, understand risks and benefits, and remember that the ultimate goal is a healthy baby.

I had been cautioned a time or two while pregnant to review my hospital bill before paying. This is laughable advice because I'm the girl who doesn't enroll in autopay for any of my bills since I like to review them first, even the ones where the dollar amount is the exact same every month. Control freak issues.

So, when the bills (yes, plural) started arriving, I would review them line by line, and with each line, I'd be more and more irate. It felt like such a scam. I hate to sound so cynical. I really do like to think most people have good intentions, but the system is so flawed.

First, I got bills for Jack's stay. Then, I got bills for my stay. I found this amusing because I'm pretty sure it was "our" stay. We're not talking a couple hundred bucks here and there, we're talking thousands of dollars, as I'm one of the many Americans with a high-deductible health plan. I probably received six bills in the mail, all contradicting each other. Then I got correction bills like, "Oopsies, you don't owe us $9,000, you only owe us $3,000." And then, "Just kidding, it's really $6,000."

Ultimately, I ended up paying. I wasn't about to break my perfect credit score, but should I be so lucky to have another child, I will most definitely ask for an overview of the charges beforehand. Health care is the only purchase we make where we don't understand the costs until after making the purchase. Imagine going to a concert and having no idea how much the tickets are and then finding out your VIP box seats cost you $7,500 each? I know, that sounds ridiculous because no one would go to a concert without knowing the ticket price. Yet, we go to the hospital to have a baby and have no clue what it costs.

One charge in particular takes the cake, though. We were charged $661 for the first thirty minutes after Jack was born, for our post-baby time in the delivery room. Felt like a steep hourly rate, but so be it. Then, the next line made my eyes bulge: $2,800 for the additional time we spent in the delivery room over the original "allotted" thirty minutes. Are you kidding me? Had I known this, I would have had us ready to go, waiting at the door by twenty-nine minutes and 30 seconds after Jack's time of birth was declared. Never once did anyone say, "If you'd like to take your time and have the nurses help you with your post-delivery clean up, it might cost you a few mortgage payments."

Do you know what they instead had the audacity to be transparent about during the hospital tour? That Justin gets as many meals as I do during our stay at no extra charge. Gee, thanks so much. His turkey sandwich and potato chips more than made up for the $2,800 dragging-your-feet-in-the-delivery-room charge.

I thought my baby-friendly hospital was the best place to be, and while I don't regret my decision, I wanted to better explore my options for the next time. After some poking around, I found a birth center in my area. According to the American Association of Birth Centers (whose tagline is "Bringing Midwifery to Main Street"), a birth center is a health care facility where the exclusive model of care is the practice of midwifery and the support of physiologic birth and newborn transition. Their motto is "Normal until Proven Otherwise", allowing for nature to run its course and providing a home-like atmosphere but still ensuring access to things like NICU services or cesarean section should the situation arise.[17]

I also decided to interview a different doctor, one who delivers at the birth center but is also more open to concepts of natural birth and natural induction techniques before jumping to pharmaceuticals. I did some research and found one whose office was closer to my house than my current practice. (Score!) I instantly fell in love with everything about the practice, including the doctor herself. It felt like a perfect fit, the same way things just feel right when you meet "the one". This is not the part of the memoir where I tell you I fell in love with the female doctor and left my husband for her, but I do think you should be a goddamn cheetah.

The lesson learned for me was know what you're getting yourself into, explore your options in your area, and stay true to your level of comfort. While I love the idea of an at-home birth, I live too far away from a medical center for comfort and wanted the reassurance of an OR and NICU nearby. I don't scoff at women who have home births or think they're hippies. On the contrary, I'm impressed and excited by them. We have to support each other and lift each other up. Your birth story doesn't have to be a fairy tale nor a nightmare. Just remember that we pay for what we get: emotionally, mentally, physically, and financially.

4

Sleeping Like a Baby, with Baby
Bedsharing

ROAD TO REBELLION

Creating our baby registry was a fun time. Now that we have a baby, I know of an activity that would be even more fun, though—following another set of first-time parents around the baby store, smiling and laughing at their pureness and naïvety as they register for items they will never actually need or use. Ah, ignorance can be such bliss, my friends.

We bought a crib. I registered for a bassinet. It wasn't even a debated topic in my mind. My baby would sleep in the bassinet next to our bed until I went back to work (when he was about four months old), and by then we'd have transitioned him to his room and his crib so I could get a good night's sleep for work. How sweet was pre-baby me? I couldn't even type that paragraph without laughing out loud and blushing a little bit at my foolishness.

Let me be clear. I was not signing up for bedsharing. I had friends who slept with their babies or kids, and the thought of it made me feel uncomfortable and unsafe. Plus, how did they ever have sex? It was a judgment-free zone on my part, but bedsharing wasn't for me.

Then, Jack was born. This teeny tiny ball of life that was relying on me to keep him safe and sound. I remember how crazy the hospital was about the baby sleeping by himself in the bassinet, which looked like a fish tank in need of a good Windexing. Anytime I put him in the bassinet, he looked absurd in there and it felt wrong. So, he was rarely in there during our two-day stay. I let him sleep on me and I'd stay awake, or while I napped I'd give him to Justin.

There is so much irony in how hard the hospital pushed things like skin-to-skin, yet they shunned co-sleeping. Remember that guy who ate blueberries, but drank brandy? Yeah, same thing here. It felt to me like they were looking at mothering in pieces instead of the focusing on the whole. There were these A.B.C. posters all over the hospital room, a cute little acronym to remind parents how babies were supposed to sleep. A: alone, B: back, C: crib. I swear if Jack could, he would have hung an F.U. poster next to every ABC one. Each time he was placed in the bassinet, he'd only sleep for a short while before waking and crying until he was picked up and held.

I was still a stickler for the rules, figuring there must be good reason for them. So, when we were home that first night, I put him in his new bassinet. He looked so little in there and so uncomfortable. Imagine going from the coolest pool float in a heated pool to lying down on the driveway. He lasted all of thirty minutes in the bassinet before waking up and crying. That first night home was long, mostly because sleeping ABC-style was not as easy as 1-2-3 for him. My nerves were frayed. Even when he did fall asleep, I'd be too paranoid to relax enough to fall asleep myself. I spent most of the night either staring at him, holding him, or nursing him. I doubt I slept more than thirty minutes total.

The second night, my bedtime rebellion started. I brought the baby lounger pillow into bed between me and Justin for Jack to sleep on. He seemed to really like the lounger. Of course he did. It was basically like taking the pool float and putting it on the driveway—a major upgrade. He slept much better, and I got maybe two hours total of sleep that night, a vast improvement from the night before. However, my guilt was through the roof as I lay next to the lounger that had all these tags on it with warnings and cautions against using the lounger in all of the ways I was using it. (Why even make the damn thing if it can only be used on the floor while baby is awake?!)

I know what you're thinking: "Toughen up, Mama. This is what newborn sleep is like." I was totally on board with sleepless nights, trust me. I love a good challenge, and I was rising to the occasion. Something deep inside me started rebelling, though, against leaving this poor little muffin by himself to sleep. It felt downright wrong.

It didn't feel wrong because my moral compass was broken. It just goes against our natural instincts as mothers. We are the ONLY mammals who sleep apart from our babies. Pause and think a moment as to what society tells us is normal. A newborn, who had only known his mother's body as a resting place (or as any place, for that matter) now has to spend hours by himself. It sounds asinine when put that way, doesn't it? You don't see a mama lion say to her cub, "Okay, you sleep in this pile of tall grass, and mommy will be just a few feet away over here."

LAURA RAFFERTY

My younger sister came to visit a few days after we'd been home from the hospital, and she watched me slowly and carefully put him into the bassinet at nighttime, while I muttered the words, "This is so fucked up." We half laughed, half cried, and she asked me, "Have you looked into a DockATot?" I looked at her with a raised eyebrow, as if to say, "She who lives the footloose and fancy-free life has a sleep solution for my five-day-old son?" She said, "Kourtney Kardashian uses one." Say no more, now I knew why she was in-the-know. My sister could probably recite every story in the tabloids, and I, on the other hand, am impressed I even knew who the Kardashians were.

In the first few months of your baby's life, money becomes no object and Amazon Prime becomes your best friend. I don't know what it is that turns new moms into frivolous spenders, but it's a real thing. I've asked around. Almost 200 dollars later, a DockATot arrived at the house. It's basically a co-sleeper where baby acts like a hot dog and the DockATot acts like a bun. (Although if you read the tags on that bad boy, it's really not meant for how I used it. Again—rebel with a cause.) We put it in the bed between us, replacing the lounger, and when I put Jack in there the first night, he snuggled in, content and cozy as could be, and my heart swelled.

A month or two later, we tried moving the DockATot from our bed into the bassinet. Justin had a get-this-baby-out-of-our-bed-before-I-accidentally-crush-him-or-swing-my-arm-into-him moment. (Have I mentioned how being a new parent can break you down from time to time?) So, I tried something different. I figured placing the DockATot IN the bassinet, three inches from my side of the bed would be fine, except I wasn't able to actually see him from where I was lying because of the bassinet siding. I burst into tears. I was so upset I couldn't stop crying. Thoughts of him not breathing or rolling over without me knowing it gave me extreme anxiety. I couldn't calm myself down, and Justin, being the understanding husband that he is (in the I-don't-understand-you-but-I love-you kind of way), got up, moved the DockATot back to where we had it previously in the bed, and we never talked about it again.

We lived like this for another three months or so: Justin, me, and Jack with the DockATot. He'd wake every three to four hours to nurse and then cozy back up in his DockATot. I was getting a manageable night's sleep and all felt right in the world until Jack started revolting against his swaddle. He wanted his arms free and spread out. This doesn't really work well in the hot dog bun for babies. So, back to the bassinet we went, sans the DockATot. (Thankfully, I could see him this way!) This time around, though, he seemed less fragile to me; and half of the time when he'd wake to nurse, I'd end up leaving him in bed with me for an extra hour because we'd both fall asleep.

We played this game for the next month or two until we did a weekend getaway to the mountains. We brought the Pack 'n Play, but not the bassinet. I felt uncomfortable with him in the Pack 'n Play while we slept because I couldn't get it as close to the bed as I could his bassinet at home. Since we were on vacation, I wanted to avoid another meltdown on my part, so I let him stay in bed with me from the beginning of the night, through the night, and it was a game-changer. I swear we both slept better (Oh, and Justin too, if anyone cares, but like, does anyone care about dad's sleep during the first year?), and from that trip onward he slept in bed with us.

Shortly after that trip, I was chatting with a girlfriend, and quietly, sheepishly, I admitted he was sleeping in our bed. "Of course he is," she said, "Where else would he sleep? My kids still sleep in our bed all of the time." She made me feel so normal. I never expected that answer from her. I had seen her children's adorable bedrooms and all the work she put into decorating them and just assumed they magically slept in there.

I did not make this decision lightly, my friends. This was the hardest area for me to be a rebel because society had me so uncomfortable with the idea of bedsharing, not to mention the look of horror from many close friends and family when I'd tell them he was in bed with me. Unfortunately, I didn't just put him in bed with us, the end, next chapter please. Instead, I spent a ton of time reading books, articles, studies (Dr. James McKenna is an underrated godsend for mamas who are scared of rebellion and need a little push), and even educating myself on sleep training. Every desperate mom needs a glimmer of hope—it just so happened that sleep training wasn't the silver lining I was looking for. The more I read, the more confident I became that bedsharing was the best thing for Jack and me and the easier it became to counter the horror of my loved ones with facts and data.

REDEFINING NORMAL

Not unlike most of the topics in this book, I knew little about baby sleep before Jack was born. I just knew that a mombie was a real thing, and that coffee and sheer willpower would be how I survived most days. Because Jack wasn't interested in solo sleeping, I found myself obsessed with knowing more about why baby sleep was such a challenge.

I have several friends who had sleep trained (Hell, my mom admitted she Ferberized me at the recommendation of her doctor), and I started following a "baby sleep trainer" on Instagram that one of my friends hired. It was a bad decision on my part, but I was desperate and curious. I found that following a baby sleep trainer is like watching a car wreck. You don't want to see it, but you can't look away. I was stunned to find out that some of these individuals are giving personalized advice on how to get your baby to sleep without ever meeting your baby! Not to mention the price tag associated with these services, hundreds of dollars in the estimates I saw.

From what I can tell, a baby sleep trainer is someone who is trained, certified (by whose definition, I'm still unsure of), or a self-proclaimed expert in tactics to get your baby to sleep by themselves and through the night. There are all sorts of antics involved often, including suggestions like standing outside your baby's door, waiting to come in and intervene only after you've listened to a "level 10" cry for three straight minutes. My mouth hit the floor.

Regardless of the antic of choice, here's what you're trying to do when you sleep train a baby: help them to connect their sleep cycles. What's a sleep cycle you ask? You mean you don't know? Kidding, I had no idea either! Apparently, we all have sleep cycles. I found sleep in general to be complex the more I learned. While you may not have known about sleep cycles, you've probably heard the term REM, even if you don't know what that means either. It's pretty simple when you break it down. Our sleep is made up of a series of cycles that are either REM or non-REM cycles. REM stands for rapid eye movement; it's the sleep we do when we're dreaming. Non-REM is when we're in a deep, restorative sleep. As we transition from cycle to cycle (for babies this can be as often as every 45-60 minutes), we stir. As adults, we're usually able to go right back to sleep[1], unless mother nature calls and we have to use the bathroom. For babies, they have a hard time transitioning and typically don't consolidate sleep cycles for the first few months. (Fun fact, babies spend more time in REM sleep than adults do, lending themselves even more so to easy arousal.)[2]

We don't train our babies to eat, walk, or talk. Sure, we HELP them with these milestones, but we're incredibly more respectful that these are developmental, and they take time. So why do we treat sleep any differently?

I'm not here to shame sleep training. I was fascinated by the concept and wondered why in the world all the energy put into sleep training didn't instead go into setting parents up for success, educating them on how sleep works, and how to safely sleep with your baby. I've equated it to dieting, and the fact that quick results sell. No one wants to sign up for a weight loss program that claims to help you lose five pounds over two months. Everyone wants the five-pounds-in-two-days diet. They all run from the "you have to make a lifestyle change" or "change your mindset" diets because who the hell wants to eat kale every day for the rest of their lives?

Aside from my gut saying, "No, no, no," there were a few data driven reasons why I didn't sleep train Jack:

- Emotional trauma: Studies have found that even once quiet after crying for mama, baby's stress hormones remain elevated for extended periods of time. They haven't learned to self soothe; they've learned to give up. If you recall, I mentioned earlier that babies this young do not have all of the brain parts necessary to regulate emotions and self soothe. Instead, what happens is they've gone silent to conserve energy, which teaches them not to seek or expect support regardless of how distressed they feel. This pretty much sealed the deal for me.[3]

- Ineffectiveness: Often, babies who are sleep trained have a regression at some point, typically during a developmental milestone or a change in schedule[4] like daylight savings (seriously the worst two weekends of the year for moms) or a vacation. The thought of doing this multiple times? Not enough thread in the world to sew my heart back together.

- Mama sleeps less: I know it's not all about me, but every so often, protecting my own sanity and well-being takes priority. I couldn't bring myself to commit to so many sleepless nights, worrying and stressing. I wasn't going to camp out with toothpicks in my eyes. I know a working mom who barely slept several nights in a row because her two-year-old was suddenly having a hard time sleeping by herself in her room (see above bullet). There were all sorts of dramatics to try to get her daughter to sleep, none of which worked, all of which created a super cranky and tired mama and toddler each morning after.

In my reading, I came across an older study from the 90s that compared U.S. middle-class families with Mayan families. When the Mayan mothers heard how the U.S. families slept separately, they were shocked and genuinely concerned for the well-being of the "neglected" U.S. babies. The concept was so foreign to them and so illogical.[5] My girlfriend's reaction when I admitted bedsharing had made me feel like I'm not crazy for feeling the same way those Mayan mamas did.

Technology is amazing. There is a crib out there that costs more than an entire bedroom set of furniture that has sensors in it to basically do what babies need (i.e., be mom). If the baby stirs, it starts rocking and hushing and even adjusts the tones of the hushing based on how fussy the baby is. That's impressive; it's okay be impressed. As baby settles down, it stops its theatrics too. It's tempting, oh it's tempting.

However, the truth is, baby fussing at night is important for their survival for two main reasons. One, it resets their breathing, which is important in the early days when sleep apnea is occurring.[6] Sleep apnea in babies is something I was unaware of, but it made me wonder if deep down moms knew this condition existed...always checking to make sure that a sleeping baby is breathing. Two, it doesn't allow them to go too long without nursing. Babies' stomachs are only so big, so breastfeeding often, even at night, is important for development.[7] Hence, the baby's proximity to mama is important when sleeping. Ready for some amazingness? Mama and baby synchronize their sleep cycles naturally when bed-sharing and breastfeeding, which allows for calm, minimal arousals between cycles for each.[8] Read: Mamas who co-sleep get more sleep, even if their baby wakes often!

It turns out I wasn't weak or a pushover but just tuned into my maternal instincts. (How validating. I'd hate to get a rap for being a softie.) We don't have to sleep train, put baby down drowsy but awake, let them cry it out, or get our babies to their own room by a certain date. Stop the "calendar parenting".[9] LOVE this term that I learned from Dr. Sears, the founding father of attachment parenting. It basically means to stop following a calendar and start following your baby's cues for changes and transitions. It is natural that our babies have a hard time falling asleep and staying asleep. It's also natural for us to be there for them.

Here's my let's-stay-friends disclosure on sleep because it's a heavily debated, highly emotional topic. If you did any of the above because you genuinely wanted to and you're happy with the results, rock on, sister. Or, if you did any of the above because you felt forced to and now your guilt is through the roof, we'll work through that in Chapter 8.

Some babies are great and can connect cycles early on and sleep alone and everyone is happy. If however that's not the case (like with Jack), the answer doesn't have to be sleep training, cry it out, or camping out. Be happy for all the proud parents who have had success, but don't compare or feel you need to follow the same path if it makes you as uncomfortable as it did me. (This is easier said than done, I know. My husband has a hard time being happy for parents whose baby just started sleeping through the night all on her own.) Rebel against it all.

I listened silently to many stories that broke my heart. Stories of mamas who let their babies cry for forty-five minutes before exhausting themselves and falling asleep. One baby soiled himself halfway through a thirty-minute cry-it-out session, which only escalated his discomfort and distress. Other stories were of mamas who were having such a hard time getting their baby to sleep alone; the baby would only sleep well in mama's bed, yet their husbands weren't on board with it. So many women resorted to sleep training because they thought they had to. We've convinced ourselves it's completely okay. We tell each other that babies cry, it's just how they communicate. Yes, that's true, but it's how they communicate stress, fear, and discomfort. Babies don't just cry to cry; there is something behind it. Fascinatingly enough, in some cultures babies rarely cry. These happen to be the same cultures that practice baby wearing, nursing on demand, and co-sleeping.[10]

Wait, if I'm at baby's beck and call, aren't I just creating a spoiled brat, and I'll never get my kid out of my bed? No, and no! It might sound like a trap, but hear me out. If you are at your baby's beck and call, you're actually creating a confident baby, one that rarely has to stress about her survival, and instead develops a healthy outlook on life. Confidence leads to independence, and independence leads to a moment where your little mini me looks at you and says, "Mom, I'm going to sleep in my own bed tonight." This moment that you never thought would happen, the one you silently prayed for so many times (or maybe not so silently), will arrive, and you'll find yourself oddly disappointed that a chaotic phase of your life is coming to a close.

WHAT WORKED FOR ME

Let me say that again, bedsharing was best for Jack and me. It may not be the best for you. In fact, I can understand if you're not sure what in the world is the best for you since there are many viewpoints on baby sleep, all of which contradict each other. You're internally conflicted on how to approach it, and the world around you is externally conflicted on how you should approach it. It's downright exhausting. (Get it?) Seriously though, I've read it all, from those who practically claim you're a terrible human being if you do anything but hold your baby like you're a kangaroo 24/7 to a fancy Manhattan pediatrician (well-respected to boot) who literally said at four months of age, put your baby in her crib at 7 p.m. and don't go back into the room until 7 a.m. Help! Who's right?

I felt this strong need, just as strong as my need for oxygen and food, to be near my baby while I was sleeping at night. As if without it, I wouldn't be able to sleep. I figured I must be a softie and immature or emotionally unstable (all, by the way, that I am never accused of) because "everyone else" has their baby sleep separately from them.

I have a truth bomb for you that I've been waiting for the perfect moment to drop, and this feels like it: "Most problems in child rearing do not have easy answers," spoken by the one and only Dr Sears.[11] If it feels too good to be true, or if it's touted as a quick fix, then know it's completely normal to feel doubtful.

Jack was not super interested in sleeping by himself, and pretty much from an early age, I'd say around four or five months, he never just randomly fell asleep. Yes, he'd go down for his naps with some help (nursing, rocking, etc.), but I would see pictures of babies who had passed out in their highchair, or sleeping in an outward-facing baby carrier, or asleep standing up in their bouncers/walkers, and I would be in awe!

SECRET WEAPONS

We all need sleep, and most importantly teeny tiny humans who are growing at a rapid pace need sleep, so I was determined to help Jack get all the rest he needed. I am NOT a baby sleep trainer, but at the risk of sounding like one, I'll share with you some of my tips and tricks that helped my little guy.

Connecting

I invented my own sleep help technique so that Jack would be well-rested during the day and coined it "connecting". (It became a real verb in our house. After a few months, my husband would ask me, "Who's connecting today, me or you?") After much research, I learned that 35–40-minute naps (i.e. waking after one sleep cycle) do not allow for some babies to get restorative sleep, which usually comes around the 60-minute mark.[12] A baby who wakes up at the 35–40-minute mark and stays up often times needs the presence of a caregiver to connect their sleep cycles (as you now know, technically they all wake briefly at this point). So around seven or eight months of age (Don't judge my foggy memory. The first year of your baby's life is a blur, and the only way you can determine timeframes is by your camera roll's date and time stamps.), when Jack went from three naps per day to two, I realized that for him, two short naps was going to make for a miserable, unrested baby boy. I decided if he can't connect his cycles, I'll connect them for him, and I started rocking Jack back to sleep when he'd wake up and let him sleep on me for the remainder of his nap. It didn't always work at first, but after a few weeks, we were golden. I even got Justin and my dad (more on him as a caregiver later on) to be able to do the same. By some blessed miracle, some days Jack would connect sleep cycles by himself and didn't need the help. However, whenever he was either teething or going through some developmental milestone, he'd consistently wake and need help. Hence, the concept of "connecting" was born in our household. It's probably one of the most relaxing things I do in parenting, and when over 50% of this book was written.

Blackout Curtains

In my desperation to get Jack to sleep longer than one sleep cycle, I stumbled upon a bit of useful information that I wish I had known sooner. Orange is not the new black. Orange is overrated, and black should stay the only black. That cute little night light I bought for the nursery? I turned it off. Turns out that for some babies, Jack being one of them, the darker the room, the better, and I'm talking pitch black. The reason being, light signals to a baby that it's daytime, or time to be awake. So if they open their eyes and see nothing, and are hopefully still sleepy, they'll have a better shot at transitioning into their next sleep cycle.

I hung on to this tidbit for dear life and did anything I could to make this work for Jack. (Desperate mama confession:

I've been known to stand in my closet with the door closed to create the darkest environment possible, rocking Jack and willing him to fall back asleep in the early hours of the morning. Sometimes I would do this for an hour, only to get him to sleep for thirty minutes more. You're not alone, Mama. I see you in that closet.)

I bought multiple sets of blackout curtains on Amazon, none of which fit my windows correctly, but I didn't care, they darkened the room tremendously. (My sister walked into my bedroom one day when she was visiting, took one look at the windows and said, "When did the handmaids get here?")

I had my husband bring duct tape and a staple gun to our Maine cottage during our summer vacation so that we could hang blackout shades in the bedroom for naps and nighttime. Not unlike many of the other shenanigans I've roped him into during parenthood, he was mortified. I wouldn't acquiesce, though, and after some convincing and a lobster roll, he committed vandalism in the name of love and slammed the staple gun into the window frames.

White Noise

Before Jack was born, we loved white noise at night and always slept with a fan going, even in the dead of winter, just for the noise. I was bummed that we'd have to break that habit when the baby was born because I'd want to be able to hear his every move. Then I learned of the 5 S's (shush, side/stomach, swaddle, sway, and suck), and "shush" saved my life.[13] I used to rock him to sleep in front of the exhaust fan in the kitchen. We bought a sound machine for the bedroom that would make you think you're in the cockpit of a fighter jet.

You may be blessed with a good sleeper in which case you probably read this chapter feeling a mix of being sorry for me and thankful you aren't me. But, I think every mama should know the following, and I wish it didn't take me six-plus months to uncover these finds:

- A sleep cycle is 35-40 minutes, and if your baby naps this long and wakes up, they may not be fully rested. They just cannot connect on their own. Like everything with babies though, there is no one size fits all, and some babies are perfectly rested and content after one of these "short naps".

- Blackout curtains are a game-changer. This may be part reality and part mental, but anything that helps my perception is just as meaningful as anything that helps my reality.

- It is OKAY if you want to sleep with your baby because your baby sleeps best that way and you're most at ease that way (and probably getting the most sleep). Just be sure to follow La Leche League's Safe Sleep Seven, which says sleeping with your baby is safe if you are:

  - A nonsmoker

  - Sober and unimpaired

- A breastfeeding mother and your baby is:

  - healthy and full-term

  - on his back

- Lightly dressed and you both are:

  - on a safe surface[14]

A note on "safe surface": See if you have better luck than I did of convincing your husband to forgo the bedframe and put the mattress directly on the floor. I know it sounds a little crazy. I'm sure you spent a good chunk of your savings when you moved in together on nice bedroom furniture, but I was just trying to ease my concerns of Jack tumbling out of bed onto the hardwood floor. A nice compromise, if you have the same results I did when broaching this subject with Daddy (Justin gave an emphatic, "Absolutely not. I have to draw the line somewhere."), is a guard rail made for the bed, or pushing your side of the bed against the wall.

There is no such thing as a bad habit when it comes to responding to our babies, especially when it comes to their sleep. Smoking cigarettes, driving without a seat belt, and eating doughnuts for breakfast—those are bad habits. Don't let me hear you shaming yourself or any other mama about the "bad habits" you've created with your baby.

Here's the thing, before I know it, Jack will be demanding his own bed with sports-themed sheets, and I'll miss these days. So yes, for a couple of years I don't get late nights out or weekend getaways with my girlfriends or cuddle sessions with my husband regularly. I had years of those things, and right now I chose to prioritize my baby over all else. Plus, once we were quarantined, we had much more time to be glued to a sleeping baby.

Do what works for you and for baby, not what works for your mother-in-law, your neighbor, your best friend, or the baby sleep trainer you follow on Instagram. Motherhood is hard enough. We need to silence all the noise in our world when it comes to our baby's sleep. Except the noise machine...keep that puppy humming for good sleep!

5

Nursing Nursing
Extended Breastfeeding

ROAD TO REBELLION

Breastfeeding: finally, a parenting topic I was totally on board with! No rebellion needed (or so I thought). "Breast is best," yeah, yeah, blah, blah, I'm all in. My number two concern going to the hospital was hoping I could breastfeed with ease (number one was getting the baby out of me safely). I'd read A LOT about it, so I felt confident I could figure it out with some help, but was still a bit worried as I'd heard many horror stories of bleeding nipples, babies who couldn't latch, boobs that couldn't produce, etc.

Once Jack was out in the real world, my focus switched to feeding him. I knew about colostrum and that for the first few days he didn't really need to eat anything, but I also knew being successful with the concept of latching was important in those first twenty-four hours of life.

I was fortunate to be in a hospital that had a phone-a-friend option for getting help with the concept of latching. Bless these beautiful souls who sign up to be lactation consultants. Honestly, they're better people than I am. Could you imagine going from room to room every day dealing with each disoriented, anxiety-ridden new mama who can't get her baby to latch and who's crying (or is that the baby crying?). These lactation consultants manage to appear almost completely oblivious to it all and just keep telling you to hold the baby like a football or a cradle and have the nipple touch the top of his mouth. "Go on, really jam it in there," they encourage. If you've never been through it before, that probably read as weird to you. If you've been there, you're crying and laughing with me.

The best is when they engage dad for the assist. My husband and I still laugh about his coaching from our lactation consultant. While I was busy holding the baby like a football (or maybe it was the cross cradle), she told Justin to take my boob and hold it like he was about to take a big bite out of a submarine sandwich. "Go on," she coaxed, "You have to make a 'breast sandwich'." Well, sports and food, my husband's love language. He nailed the breast sandwiches, and thankfully Jack's natural born instincts kicked in, and Justin got him to latch on the first try.

We did it! By the time we left the hospital, Jack was a breastfeeding fool, and I had porn star boobs. (Really, I did. I remember looking at myself topless in the hospital room bathroom mirror feeling like I must be looking in one of those fun house mirrors. There is no way those beach balls could be mine.) They're not kidding when they say, you'll just "know" when your milk comes in. It definitely enters the room like a whore walking into church.

A few weeks later, I was feeling cocky and confident as I strolled into Jack's follow-up doctor's appointment because he'd been breastfeeding like a champ. Then, I got thrown a curveball. Come to find out, there are rules within rules. Breast might be best, but only if it's every two to three hours. If you ask the AAP, breast is only best until baby is twelve months old[1], or according to the WHO until baby is twenty-four months old[2]. I'll share more about it in Redefining Normal. How in the world are new moms supposed to keep all this straight when we can barely keep our eyes open?

This is before I started censoring myself with my doctors. I was still young and naïve at this visit and hadn't embraced the mama white lies. So, when asked how frequently he nursed, I answered truthfully and said, "About every 75 minutes to every 2 hours." The nurse practitioner paused from taking notes, looked up at me, and said, "Don't let him abuse you. See if he'll take a pacifier." I was so deflated! Here I was, thinking I was doing such great things for my baby, and now I had to slow down with how frequently he was nursing? I didn't feel abused, but obviously she must know what she's talking about. (I could have used a little angel on my shoulder saying, "instinct versus instruction", to combat this devil with horns in front of me.)

Mamas, how many times has that happened to you? You think you're doing the right thing, or at least everything feels right, and suddenly you're told otherwise? I went home and called those beautiful souls (Yes, they give you a hotline for the lactation consultants when you leave the hospital. Talk about gluttons for punishment!) and told them how frequently I was feeding and what the nurse practitioner said to me, and the lactation consultant said:

"So, he's gaining weight appropriately?"

"Well, yes."

SECRET WEAPONS

Nursing Tank Tops

Investing in some nursing tank tops was a game changer. Invest might be a strong word; gather your couch cushion change and you should be just fine. I think I spent about thirty USD on a set of three, but I wore them religiously, washing them on the delicate cycle and hang-drying to preserve them. I treated them better than some women treat their wedding gowns, but they are so convenient. Just a little unclick and out comes the utter. Because nursing made me like a furnace 24/7, rarely did I need to wear anything else. On the occasional chilly day, though, I would throw on a zip-up sweater so that it was still easy access. Ah, my maternity leave uniform, worn with pride.

Breastfeeding Tracking App

Breastfeeding tracking app. Jack, my boobs, and I contently lived in harmony around the clock, and I used a handy dandy app on my phone for the first few weeks to track when he fed and what boob he fed from. It was the new-age version of the old "pin on the blouse" trick.

"And the feeding schedule is working for you and him?"

"Well, yes."

"Then it sounds like you're doing everything just right for you two. Keep doing exactly what you're doing."

There it is. I quickly got my confidence back and remembered there is no one-size-fits-all, which is why breastfeeding has a place in this book. I LOVED breastfeeding, but I rebelled against any structure provided to how you should "properly" breastfeed. The lactation consultant was spot on...keep doing what works for you two. Only you and your baby truly know what the best pace is for you.

In fact, not only is it okay to frequently nurse in those early days, but it's also common and has an appropriate name: cluster feeding. I will never forget my first experience with cluster feeding. When Jack was barely one month old, I was excited to watch the live version of the movie *Dumbo*. I'm not sure I thought through the tragic mom and baby separation at the time I picked out the film, but I never made it that far into the movie...which was probably for the best. I avoided unnecessarily activating the postpartum waterworks. When Jack fell asleep, we turned it on. Unlike prior naps, he woke up incredibly fussy after fifteen minutes. I tried a few different things before I realized he wanted to nurse again! I let him latch, he nursed, and he unlatched. But, within a few minutes he was fussy again. We latched on the other boob this time, he drank, unlatched, and was still discontent. At this point the well was starting to run dry, and I was sweating a little bit because it didn't appear like he was going to slow down any time soon. As cute as he was, he was starting to resemble a starved madman who couldn't be satiated. His frustration only grew at the realization that the supply was running low, which was increasing my stress levels to near hysteria. Finally, after ninety minutes of nursing him, practically continuously, he gave pause. The only words I could utter were, "Someone get me the graham cracker box," and I silently ate four sheets of graham crackers and drank two large glasses of water, completely famished. I can never think of Dumbo or graham crackers without remembering that night.

About one month into my motherhood journey, I started pumping. This was another one of those breastfeeding rules I followed, but because it came from the beautiful soul lactation consultants, I felt good about this rule. They told me to wait about a month to start pumping to allow my milk supply to regulate. So, I did. It was another proud moment, watching those bottles fill up. Real talk, though, the sensation of the pump took a little getting used to. It was intense at first and did not feel like it does when baby nurses. It's more like a vacuum pulsing on your nipples. It sounds intimidating, but you'll be used to it in no time. Pretty much like everything else in motherhood, intimidating at first, but you get used to it. And, are you ready for this? I read SEVERAL books about breastfeeding, and never once did I come across this fascinating fact. Ladies, if you've never pumped before, I hope you're sitting down for this mind blower. There is more than one hole in your nipple. Yup! There are actually many, like at least six or seven, by my count. When the milk comes out, it looks like some beautiful fountain in an Italian piazza. I feel like it's breastfeeding's best kept secret, and one you must know about! No need for alarm the first time you see multiple streams. It's completely normal.

While I took to pumping like a champ, Jack was a bit more resistant. He refused the bottle. I know what you're thinking, I was too impatient, give it time. But, he refused the bottle pretty much up until we stopped offering him a bottle, around eight months of age. I did all the tricks. I made sure I was nowhere in sight or scent when Justin would give him the bottle. I had multiple people try giving him the bottle, so he wasn't only expecting Justin. Yes, I even tried different bottles. I tried probably six or seven different bottles before I came to terms with the fact that it's not the bottle nor the bottle giver, it's the baby.

Like a good soldier, for twelve weeks I pumped once per day, and someone gave him a bottle once per day until my first day back to work. It was a sad day when I had to go back to work (probably the biggest understatement of my life) for so many reasons, but one of them being that it meant nursing on demand wasn't going to be our daily routine anymore, and I'd have to pump more regularly. None of that sounded enjoyable, as I was already beside myself with grief to be separated from Jack. But, it was even less enjoyable because I had to find time three times per day to sit in a conference room, pump, store my milk in a communal fridge, and clean my pump parts in the communal sink after each time. I'd do a walk of shame down the hallway with my special zip-locked bags filled with milk.

I would lament and laugh about the woes with other moms who had pumped at work. I had coworkers tell me they had switched to formula because pumping was just too much work, and their kids grew up just fine, but I wasn't going to quit that easily. I was certain that my baby would benefit from breast milk, and I wasn't even close to ready to give up our nursing sessions when I was home. I was happy to continue pumping and nursing, with my eye on an arbitrary finish line of twelve months old.

I felt that way right up until Jack's first birthday was approaching. Before Jack was born, I would go around saying, "Six months is nonnegotiable, so help me God, even if my nipples are falling off. I will nurse this boy until he's six months old. Nine months is ideal, and twelve months would make me a super star." What was behind this reasoning? To give it to you straight: a lot of ignorance and a little bit of guidance from the so-called experts. I picked six months because that's when he'd start real food, then nine months because I heard that's the point when they should start to pick up on the eating (hardy har, more on that later), and then twelve months because, well, who nurses past twelve months? Only weirdos, right? So, I was feeling confident in my twelve-month ultimate goal despite conflicting information from AAP and WHO on the appropriate stop date.

Twelve months might sound like a long time to a new mom. I know it did to me. I lost all rights and privileges to my body many moons ago when I got pregnant with Jack. Since then, I've either been a baby-building machine or a baby-feeding machine. He takes all the good stuff, and leaves me what's left behind, often in the form of cellulite and dark eye circles. There's only so much physical abuse a mama can take before she waves the white flag and declares, "Pour me a glass of wine," or "Bring me coffee."

Before you start thinking otherwise, I didn't drink an ounce of alcohol from about a week before I took my positive pregnancy test until over a month after Jack was born. Nowhere in this book are you going to find me telling you to be a rebel and get smashed while either pregnant or nursing. (Or, for that matter, even if not nursing. Time to be a responsible adult. There is a small child in your care.) Those days are behind you, so I hope you enjoyed them when you had them.

I did A LOT of research to determine if I could have the occasional glass of wine (1-2 glasses, at most) without having to pump and dump or buy overpriced breast milk test strips and examine my expressed milk like I was back in a high school science lab. It took me a while to get comfortable enough to enjoy a glass of wine without worrying Jack would have permanent damage. Most advice reads like, "Yes, on occasion you can drink alcohol, but in general we recommend you abstain." Thank you for the lackluster answer, but I'm obviously looking to you for advice because abstaining for the prior ten plus months was enough abstinence for me.

After much digging, looking for real studies and legitimate data, I was able to take the dust off my corkscrew without feeling uneasy. My findings were that within reason, it's perfectly fine. You don't have to waste time pumping and dumping. An occasional glass of wine or beer is not off limits, but if you want to be uber conservative, wait an hour or two after a drink before you nurse. More on this in Redefining Normal.

With regards to coffee, I had a cup during pregnancy maybe two or three times per month. I wasn't the biggest coffee drinker before getting pregnant. Instead, I enjoyed green tea daily. However, once I got pregnant, simply the idea of green tea turned me green. As a result, on the weekends I'd have a cup of joe sometimes. I was pregnant with my first baby, meaning I could still sleep whenever I wanted to. I'm pretty energetic as it is, so exhaustion wasn't something I was often faced with.

When Jack was born, holy wow, those first few weeks can zap you good. My once per weekend cup turned into a once per day cup, but I would make the pot three parts regular, four parts decaf. You know, because the mom guilt of having fully caffeinated coffee would be a worse feeling than the sharp and dull pain behind my eyes from only sleeping forty-five minutes in two days.

REDEFINING NORMAL

Warning: This section is one big giant nerd emoji. It's by far the dorkiest Redefining Normal in the entire book, so of course I think it's the coolest section. I recommend you pause, grab a cup of (guilt-free) coffee, and be ready to have your mind blown!

Let's start with the baby binge sessions in those early days. In the moment, cluster feeding can make you feel trapped and under the gun, so it's helpful if you go into it knowing how amazing cluster feeding actually is. Listen to your baby. They're trying to increase your milk supply for an impending growth spurt, and somehow your baby just knows that the only way to do that is to nurse often. Breast milk production is a total supply and demand system.[3] How frigging amazing is that? Your tiny bundle of joy has the natural instinct to increase your milk supply. Talk about survival tactics! When cluster feeding comes knocking on your door, know that nothing is wrong with you or your baby. Just hunker down, grab your graham crackers, and find a movie (anything other than Dumbo) to distract you from the marathon nursing of cluster feeding.

With regards to alcohol consumption, the science is pretty interesting, so humor me and listen while I geek out. Alcohol passes into breast milk in approximately the same concentrations as it does into your blood stream. Studies have shown that level of concentration would expose the baby to 5-6% of what the mother ingested, and that's assuming she nurses at the peak of when the alcohol is at the highest concentration (usually 30-60 minutes after consumption). Even if a nursing mom has two drinks in a relatively short period of time and then nurses her baby at peak, the blood alcohol level of the child would be 0.0025%, which is roughly 3% of mom's blood alcohol level[4] —very small.

It's worth noting that alcohol seems to slow your down your let down[5] (let down is simply your milk releasing through your nipples). I suppose that makes sense. In general alcohol slows down most things in us (think: racing thoughts and hand-eye coordination). So, don't panic, you're not dried up. Although you may produce less because alcohol does cause dehydration, and water is helpful in keeping up your milk supply.

Dr. Jack Newman, MD, from the International Breastfeeding Centre in Canada said, "Prohibiting alcohol is another way we make life unnecessarily restrictive for breastfeeding mothers."[6] Also, I love the way one of the studies that I read ended, "In conclusion, special recommendations aimed at lactating women are not warranted. Instead, lactating women should simply follow standard recommendations on alcohol consumption."[7] In other words, be a responsible adult. Follow guidelines for moderate drinking.

Caffeine: Coffee is something the experts are much more straightforward about. According to La Leche League, we can have up to 300 mg of caffeine while nursing.[8] We're talking a large coffee (about 20 oz) before you're in the danger zone, which means the roughly eight ounces of caffeinated coffee I was consuming was way below the threshold. I'm a sucker for extra credit, so I kept my pot at a 3:4 ratio.

In all of my caffeine research, I repeatedly read to be on the lookout for irritable behavior in baby, or a hard time falling/ staying asleep, especially in the early months.[9] While, yes, there are about a million reasons that might be the case besides your cup of joe, it is something to consider if you're indulging in a latté regularly. However, for the most part, you should be in the clear and can take the toothpicks out of your eyes and put a mug in your hand.

While we know breastfeeding isn't a one-size-fits-all answer, I checked in with the experts on their recommendations for how long to breastfeed. The American Academy of Pediatrics recommends "...exclusive breastfeeding for about 6 months, followed by continued breastfeeding as complementary foods are introduced, with continuation of breastfeeding for 1 year or longer as mutually desired by mother and infant."[10]

Since I'm leery of the United States parenting guidelines from some of my other research, I decided to see what the rest of the world was doing on this topic too. The World Health

Organization recommends "...mothers worldwide to exclusively breastfeed infants for the child's first six months to achieve optimal growth, development and health. Thereafter, they should be given nutritious complementary foods and continue breastfeeding up to the age of two years or beyond".[11]

Two years or beyond? Come to find out, humans just recently stopped breastfeeding at such early ages of one year or less.[12] Recently is relative to the fact that we've been around for millions of years. The AAFP (American Academy of Family Physicians) states that it has been estimated that a natural weaning age for humans is between two and seven years.[13] Did you hear that? The minimum was age two. MINIMUM. My mind was blown, and I had to dig more into this.

This statement stems from anthropologist Kathy Dettwyler's research. She suggests that the normal and natural duration of breastfeeding for modern humans falls between 2.5 years at a minimum and about 7 years at a maximum. Up until the last 100 years or so, natural term breastfeeding was a cultural norm. She did a ton of research on non-human primates, as well, since they're our closest thing to family in the animal kingdom. Dettwyler says, "Many primates wean their offspring when they are erupting their first permanent molars. This occurs around five-and-a-half to six years in modern humans around the same time as achievement of adult immune competence suggesting that throughout our recent evolutionary past the active immunities provided by breastmilk were normally available to the child until about this age."[14]

Should we consider updating our terminology then? Is it more appropriate that "premature weaning" is the term for those who stop before age one, instead of "extended breastfeeding" being used to describe anyone who nurses past age one? Would perspectives change? Would behavior evolve? Could we then tell all of our noisy family members to go skip rocks so we can carry on with our developing toddler?

I couldn't help myself; I created this little bonus section for you on some more nursing awesomeness. I present to you:

The Roundup of the Coolest Breastfeeding Tidbits

1. *Breast crawl video (https://www.youtube.com/watch? v=b3oPb4Wd ycE)* [15]: *I know it sounds like a dance move, but this is the coolest phenomenon I've seen when it comes to breastfeeding! If you put a baby on your chest directly after birth, he'll crawl (more like shimmy) his way to your nipple and attempt to latch. Just watch the video; I can't do it justice in words. It's completely bush league in production, but it is all things beautiful and awe-invoking.*

2. *When you hear a crying baby, you leak. If this isn't PROOF that mothers are built to respond to their baby when the baby is in distress[16], and that NATURE provides breastmilk to soothe, I don't know what else will convince you. If you're not convinced, you should probably just stop reading the book now and put it in your library's donation bin.*

3. *This one rocked my world. Studies have shown that the breastfeeding process is a two-way street. You're giving the baby milk, and her saliva is giving your body signals as to any sickness...and the number of antibodies will increase in your breast milk![17]*

4. *Caloric content changes as baby gets older. Worried about how many ounces to give the baby and when to increase? Worry no more! The caloric content will adjust as your baby gets older, even accounting for things like growth spurts.*[18]

5. *Breastfeeding is a form of birth control. Mamas have less than a 2% chance of getting pregnant again during the first six months of exclusively breastfeeding.*[19] *This could backfire on the other end if you're still breastfeeding after a year yet want to get pregnant. They say it's your baby's way of telling you they're not ready for a younger sibling...yet.*

6. *Snack Attack: Breastfeeding requires roughly an additional 500 calories*[20] *which means an extra two to three snacks per day. YUM! Note, I hesitate to quote these generic calorie requirements, so take it with a grain of salt and listen to your hunger.*

7. *Breastfeeding prevents common female diseases. Studies have shown that nursing moms receive protection against pre-menopausal breast cancer (especially those who practice extended breastfeeding), ovarian cancer, and osteoporosis. One study estimated that our current high rates of breast cancer in western countries would be reduced by almost half if we increased our lifetime duration of breastfeeding.*[21] *Save the ta-tas!*

While I just told you all the wonders of breastfeeding, I'd be remiss if I didn't share the other side of the story which involves cracked nipples, clogged ducts, and conditions like thrush and mastitis. We're not going to spend much time here because I was fortunate to not have experienced too many rough patches, but it's only fair that going into this breastfeeding journey you know the good, the bad, and the ugly, and you're aware of warning signs to be on the lookout for.

Cracked or bleeding nipples: I know women who are literally wiping transferred blood off their baby as they nurse. This can be incredibly stressful and psychologically impact a woman's ability to nurse. This is not to be confused with rusty pipe syndrome. Rusty pipe syndrome is when a small amount of blood enters a mama's breast milk and turns it pinkish or rusty in color. It goes away after a few weeks and causes no harm to your baby and is completely internal; there are no external cuts/cracks.[22]

The rawness you'll feel in your nipples at the beginning of your nursing journey needs some TLC. I was constantly applying nipple balm throughout the day to help combat it. Find a nipple balm that is safe for baby to consume so you don't have to stress about having just applied some and then hearing the "feed me" cry. The first month (or two, just keeping it real) can be a challenge for your girls to get adjusted. This is common, but I swear your nipples will toughen up and you'll barely feel anything in due time. Remember Vince Vaughan's crazy sister-in-law from Four Christmases? Well, I wouldn't take an ounce of parenting advice from her, but she was spot on when she said, "Maybe at first, but the nipples get tough," to inquiring Reese Witherspoon. Hang in there!

Clogged ducts: I've been here several times, and it's important to note that on the way down (i.e. when you're weaning) these are common. You'll know when you have one. It'll feel like you were shot in the boob with a BB gun, and there is now a red-hot golf ball lodged in your breast. In fact, Rudolph's nose wasn't the only thing that was round, red, and hot on Jack's second Christmas Eve. The night before Christmas, when all through the house, not a creature was stirring, not even my blouse. My sister was visiting from out of town, so I was elated to be physically present with someone other than my son, husband, and parents (No disrespect, but quarantine life could get lonely at times.), and I went to bed happy and peaceful. So happy and peaceful that I slept on my stomach, an old favorite position of mine. It just so happened that Jack slept really well through that night, barely waking to nurse. Combine the two (sleeping on breasts + not expressing breasts for hours) and you get a clogged duct!

I woke up and knew right away, for this wasn't my first clogged duct. I quickly went into remediation mode: hot wash cloth, breast pump, and some elbow grease for a serious deep tissue massage on the culprit. I had to take my pump out of retirement, dust it off, and I hung upside down on my bed (the stockings were hung and so were my boobs) because I had read that nursing (or pumping) from different angles can help work out the blockage. There I was, manhandling my boob with brute-like force while my sister held my pump. I'm sure she mentally noted that motherhood wasn't all baby cuddles and giggles.

You may be inclined to avoid nursing/pumping when the boob has a clogged duct, but fight the urge! Let baby feed on the boob with the clogged duct; the only thing that is going to fix the issue is to bust through the clog, so sucking, heat, and massage all help.[23] Plus, remember there are several other ducts in that boob, so just because one is clogged, doesn't mean that ta-ta is useless.

Because it was Christmas Eve, I wanted to shake this as fast as possible so I could get back to being jolly. I went a step further and added in some natural remedies. I had remembered hearing that raw garlic has antibiotic-like properties, so I swallowed six garlic clove halves (yes, three garlic cloves in total) like they were vitamins. It wasn't that bad going down, but I never thought far enough ahead to the coming out part. Suffice it to say, I basically could have serenaded my family with my toots to the tune of "Jingle Bells" the next day.

Mastitis: an infection that is oftentimes a clogged duct gone mad (hence my holiday panic), or it could result from an open cut on the nipple, weakened immune system, or even high stress or fatigue.[24] (See why it's so important to take care of yourself?) If you're unsuccessful in treating a clogged duct, and it turns into mastitis, you'll want to call you OB-GYN. I remember my doctor telling me to call right away if I felt like I had the flu— chills, fever, nausea—and a prescription would be called in for an antibiotic. All of my shenanigans in treating my clogged ducts thankfully spared me from ever having experienced mastitis.

Thrush: I have not had it, but I had a girlfriend who had it and said it was like a never-ending game of ping pong. She and her son were just passing it back and forth. It's essentially a yeast infection (the same type that you could get vaginally)[25], and yeast infections can be super pesky when trying to get rid of it. You'll notice signs such as burning or itching when you nurse, and you'll notice signs on your baby if you see white patches in her mouth or a fussiness when latching or nursing.[26] Again, don't mess around, call the doctor.

What Worked for Me

If the title of the chapter didn't give it away, and you didn't follow my foreshadowing on the last several pages, then here's your spoiler alert. When Jack turned one year old, yes, we had a smash cake, we wore party hats, and we celebrated his beautiful life, but we didn't stop nursing. I did not cut him off, and he didn't stop. The only thing that stopped that day was my calendar parenting. I no longer put a deadline on nursing, and I followed Jack's lead.

I'm embarrassed by my limited thinking as I type this, but know better do better, right? I can remember scoffing at these "weird" moms who nurse their babies over twelve months, perturbed by stories like "he just goes right up to her and pulls down her shirt, nurses quickly, and then keeps playing." If you are of the mindset I was, stop for a minute and ask yourself this question: Is that really any different than the little toddler who's running around like a madman, pauses for a second to take a swig of his juice box, and then carry on? You know which mom we should be judging? (Trick question. NEITHER—remember this is a judgement-free zone.) Real talk—a sugary juice box is the less nutritional option for a toddler yet the one that we all think is perfectly fine and don't bat an eyelash at. Meanwhile, the mom who still nurses throughout the day after her child is one year old is thought of as some weird hippie.

I became one of those weirdo women who practiced extended

nursing. Extended nursing is a term I hate but willingly use because it's widely recognized, albeit it's such an arbitrary concept. A mama who nurses past four minutes, four days, four weeks, four months, or four years may all have considered themselves having practiced extended nursing. Conversely, you could argue that a mama who nurses less than four minutes, four days, four weeks, four months, or four years prematurely weans. It's all about perspective, and neither mama is weird at all; they're just following their instinct versus instruction.

During my reading, I came across a term that broke my heart: closet nursing. It's used to describe women who do continue nursing well past age one but do so in their privacy of their own home, keeping it a secret, and in some cases outright lying about the fact they are still nursing.[27] As I read this account, shaking my head, I realized, "Wait a minute. I'm closet nursing too!" I'm living through a pandemic, quarantined at home, and the only people who see me nurse my toddler are my husband and my parents. I was mad at myself and vowed that when the opportunity presented itself in conversation, I would openly discuss that Jack is still nursing. How can we ever change the behavior and the mindset if we don't put it out there?

I've seen women sheepishly admit to extended breastfeeding, and I've watched the other women around her give her a sympathetic look...like this poor thing, she can't possibly want to be doing this, but she is just too weak or doesn't have the heart to cut off her baby. It doesn't even cross people's mind that MAYBE she's fine with it. Maybe it gives her peace of mind that her baby is still drinking the magical milk for mental, emotional, and physical development. Maybe mama loves the bonding experience, the opportunity to just slow it down for a few minutes and relax (Hello, prolactin and oxytocin!), and soak in her muffin's scent. However, because us mamas admit it like dogs with our tails between our legs, it's assumed we're doing it under duress.

I know what you're thinking, but what about the teeth? How the hell did she prevent biting and nipping? Did she just grin and bear it? While I've got some good grit and a high tolerance of pain (Did you hear that, Kathy?), I was not about to have my poor nipples bitten for months and months. Jack popped his first two teeth when he was four months old, but I can count on one hand how many times he bit me. The first time I reacted so instinctually and yelped loudly. I scared both of us and he started to cry, and he didn't bite me again for many months. The next time he did, he was much older, and I reacted the same way. This time I could tell he was torn between whether we were playing a game or whether he did something wrong. He ended up determining it was the latter, burst into one of the most dramatic crying sessions to date, and never bit me again.

I don't have a unicorn baby, mamas. I've read countless accounts of mamas who had similar situations. If we react with our natural instinct, baby will sense that biting wasn't the right thing to do. I even read a story about a woman who did yelp and pulled her baby away, and even though that worked, and her baby didn't bite her again, she felt so guilty about it. When she had her second baby, she tried to grin and bear it, and instead used calming words to articulate to her baby that was a no-no. Guess how that worked out for her? Baby never got the message, the biting continued, and she eventually quit nursing because she couldn't take it.[28] I don't mean to keep bringing us back to our mammalian cousins here, but so many mammals nurse their toothed-up babies, and they don't have special nipples. They just lay down the law the same way, and life is good.

It's almost impossible for me to talk about what worked for me with breastfeeding without talking about bed-sharing. You can absolutely do one without the other, but when you do both, there is such harmony. "Nursing him to sleep is creating a bad habit." Is it? I'm pretty sure that if I didn't nurse Jack to sleep at night, I'd be rocking, reading, and wrestling this madman for hours. I know I sound like a broken record, but breastfeeding, bedsharing mamas get more sleep. Let me say it again for those in the back. You will get more sleep, Mama! There is no waking up, puttering down the hallway, nursing and/or shushing back to sleep, only to do it again in a couple of hours. Especially an older baby or toddler who is teething, frequent night awakenings due to discomfort are completely common. Instead, when you bed-share, you snuggle up, half awake, make sure your baby has access to your nipple, and drift back to sleep.

While daytime nursing slowly becomes less frequent as your child gets older and starts eating more solid foods there is nothing cuter than a milk drunk toddler. When they unlatch and walk away it's like watching your best friend get up from a bar stool after one too many martinis. You look at them with so much love in your eyes, hoping they don't stumble into the wall, and you pray like hell they won't pass out and ruin your chances of getting late night pizza.

Let's breastfeed for as long as we and our babies mutually enjoy it. For some of us that might be two days, for others that might be two years. If you join me in nursing nursing, know you are not a weirdo, but a beautiful nurturing mama.

6

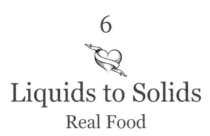

Liquids to Solids
Real Food

ROAD TO REBELLION

"He's small for gestation, so we're going to have to test his glucose levels every ninety minutes for the first twenty-four hours. If they dip below normal, we'll need him to nurse within fifteen minutes, otherwise we'll have to give him formula. Once he goes twenty-four hours within normal range, he'll be in the clear."

This was all thrown at me within hours of giving birth. I was so focused on preparing for what could go wrong during the actual birth part, that I realized I was inadequately prepared for what could go wrong afterwards. Head spinning, I simply nodded at the nurses. Just like that, Jack was sucked into the world of consumption obsession. I'm not trying to minimize the importance of food; I know it's literally required for survival. Having been raised by a full-blooded Italian, I've seen firsthand how the intense focus on intake can be a bit too much.

As you know, Jack's birth weight was what they coin "small for gestation" because on the day he was born, I was one day shy of forty-one weeks pregnant, and his six-pound, six-ounce (adorable) frame didn't fit in the normal range on their charts. By their standards, he should have been bigger. If you ask my

OB-GYN, it's because my placenta called it quits sometime in the last few weeks of pregnancy. Apparently, my OB-GYN didn't share that message with the hospital, so the hospital was looking at his birth weight with tunnel vision, and being concerned, required him to take this glucose test every ninety minutes (which I later found out was an additional line item on my nice, long hospital bill).

I wasn't prepared for this, didn't even know it was a thing. I barely digested (pun intended) the disclaimer spewed at me by the nurses. The next thing I knew, his little heel was being pricked, and we were all holding our breath as we waited for the digital reader to show us a number. I don't remember what it was, but I remember he passed the test, and I passed a sigh of relief.

The nurses said mother's body heat helps keep the levels up, so do plenty of skin-to-skin contact...except, of course, when we have to sleep. Then we have to wrap that poor muffin in his swaddle and put him in his lonely bassinet. So ass backwards these rules are! Skin-to-skin was no chore for me; I happily snuggled him every waking minute. Despite my efforts, one of the next few times the nurses came in to check, his level read one number below the lowest range of the safety zone. One freaking number off, and all hell broke loose. Immediately I had to try to get him to breastfeed, and one of the hospital staff members had to witness him drinking. Oh, okay, no pressure or anything. If it didn't happen within fifteen minutes, they were going to give him formula. My heart sank. Formula wasn't in my plans. I was adamant I would exclusively breastfeed, and my baby was not going to drink any dairy products while doing so. I asked if there were any plant-based formulas available or milk donations available. The nurse looked at me like I was some bougie snob and basically told me no. She gave some short remark about not recommending soy-based formula at this age (as if the milk intended for a baby cow was much better) and that all the milk donations were frozen and wouldn't be thawed in time for Jack's fifteen-minute countdown.

Try as I did, I couldn't get Jack to nurse. I mean, of course I couldn't, there was NOTHING to drink but a little colostrum. I'm sure the stress of having to perform on command was preventing both of us from successfully completing this ridiculous task. So, in comes the lactation specialist with a tiny bottle of formula, and she took Jack from me and placed a few drops in his mouth.

I tried to stay calm. One sip of formula wasn't going to ruin him, but I was saddened. I didn't feel ownership over my baby. It felt like I was on trial to purchase him from the hospital and my future as his "owner" was looking bleak. Thankfully every test thereafter, he registered acceptable glucose levels, and within twenty-four hours he no longer had to be monitored.

By day four of Jack's life, his weight had exceeded his birth weight, which is often unheard of so soon after birth, as many babies take one to two weeks to get back up to their birth weight due to the loss of fluids and the learning curve of having to actually feed yourself (no more umbilical cord to do all of the work). He quickly hopped up to the 40th to 50th percentile in weight and has stayed there ever since. Initially, I tracked this obsessively, but over time I chilled out, or at least thawed a bit.

Chilling out is still something I'm working on in general; see Chapter 9. A real triumph for me was when I told my OB-GYN at my six-week postpartum appointment that Jack was over ten pounds. She was impressed and gave me kudos for a job well done. What mama doesn't love a little praise for her mothering?

I should have learned a valuable lesson in the hospital with all of Jack's glucose tests: Lower your expectations on how your baby's feeding journey unfolds. Six months later though, those glucose tests and the formula-tasting were distant memories, and I strode into kitchen with my head held high, confident that my puréed sweet potatoes would be a bigger hit than even my green bean casserole on Thanksgiving (and EVERYONE has seconds of that taste of heaven).

Just like everything I had read advised, I waited six months to give Jack "real" food. I baked and puréed sweet potatoes one weekend around his half-birthday. With our phone cameras ready to capture that first spoonful, Justin and I fed Jack this orange wonder. I had zero expectations that he would eat much of it, realizing this would be his first experience with real food and it would seem foreign. It went surprisingly well in that he actually swallowed several spoonfuls. He made the most adorable faces. Sometimes happy, sometimes curious, and more than once a face that look like we just fed him feces.

I decided I'd make all my own baby food. Not only was it cost-effective, but then I could ensure it was natural and that it actually tasted like the foods (since part of this whole progression to solids was initially about acquiring tastes and preferences). If you've ever tasted most jarred baby food, it

BARELY tastes like what it's touted as, most likely because of the attempt made to give it a shelf life. I proceeded to make so many purées, froze them in little ice cube trays, microwaved them individually for each meal, got Jack to consume one or two spoonfuls, and then ended up throwing most of them out or finishing them for him. Admittedly, even if he didn't think so, some of them were absolutely delicious.

The next month or so was a trip (roller coaster ride is probably more like it) along the rainbow, offering him fruits and vegetables of all colors and tastes, none of which he was overly thrilled with, many of which after a taste or two he was done. Suffice it to say, we never heard him say, "My compliments to the chef."

I schemed solutions to the disinterest in purées. First, I blamed it on the spoon. Jack was always taking the spoon in his hand and flipping it around, inserting the end with no food on it into his mouth. I went out of my way (in that my internet search and purchase took a total of twenty minutes instead of three), to find two-sided spoons...so he could flip and dip. I thought this would encourage him to eat since no matter which end of the spoon he put into his mouth, there would be food on it. Total waste of money and twenty minutes.

Then I thought maybe he would eat the purées from those trendy squeeze pouches because he would be in full control. Even at this tender age, I could see my little protégé was transforming into a control freak just like mama. So, I bought reusable pouches and showed him how to squeeze and suck, but he was more interested in tossing them over his highchair and watching them land on the floor.

After several weeks, a dozen or so foods, and a couple of useless purchases, I had a light bulb moment that the problem must be my blender. It was a basic blender, one I had owned for a decade. I convinced myself that if I had a fancy high-speed blender, I could get the consistency creamier, and the texture would be more appealing. Oh, what's that you say? My faulty logic was louder than the blender blades? Well, smarty pants, where were you when I needed someone to hold up the mirror to me?

I decided to approach Justin about buying a Vitamix. That might sound ridiculous. I more than adequately contributed financially to our household, and I shouldn't have to request permission to upgrade a kitchen appliance. But, a $600 blender? How insane does that sound? I had been wanting one forever for my smoothies but could never justify the cost. As we've talked about, money oddly becomes no object when you are a new mom trying to survive.

I finally worked up the courage to ask him, and much to his credit, he didn't burst out laughing in my face. He actually let me use some gift cards he had to buy a Vitamix and threw in the single-serve cups for my smoothies. Is he a keeper or what? Hopeful that this would be a game changer, I was quickly proven otherwise when the first purée made by the Vitamix was just as uninteresting to Jack as the prior ones. I was, however, incredibly satisfied with the consistency of my smoothies.

Around the same time, a friend of my sister came over with her son who was days apart in age from Jack. She asked if I minded if she used my microwave to heat up her son's meal, to which I replied of course not. The next thing I know, she whips out a lunch tote with all these food containers. I started to wonder if she brought dinner for her and her husband, worried she didn't like my party spread of snacks. In my mind, there was no way her baby was going to eat all of that. It was more food than Jack consumed in a day, forget about one meal. Yet, he did! No fuss, right off the spoon. Patiently waiting for each mouthful, no mess.

I was talking with a few girlfriends when I was at least one month into the solid food journey with Jack. One of the girlfriends had a daughter just a couple months younger than Jack, and she was sharing how her daughter loves to eat everything, even avocado spooned right out of the shell. At this point in my motherhood journey, I was noticing a pattern that Jack wasn't exactly your average Joe, and instead he balked at most modern baby "norms", like bottle feeding, crib sleeping, and puréed foods. When asked how Jack was doing with food, I admitted, "All right, he doesn't seem to really love most of what I give him," visions of my sister's friend's baby gobbling up butternut squash and baby oatmeal taunting me in my head. I then went on to tell them the only food he gets excited about is if I am eating an apple. He likes to take turns handing it back and forth with me, and he'll suck on the juice when it's his turn with the apple.

My other girlfriend, who has two older toddler boys, said, "He's telling you something. Have you heard of baby-led weaning?" Of course, I had not heard of baby-led weaning. Add it to the list of seven thousand things I had no idea about before motherhood. Resilience becoming my new middle name, instead of being discouraged at my lack of information, I was hopeful this little nugget would be the key to success for mealtime with Jack. Off to the library I went, ready to learn about baby-led weaning, and I was instantly intrigued.

REDEFINING NORMAL

This was refreshing. As of current, all the acronym organizations are on the same page as to when to start solids, both WHO[1] and AAP[2] recommend exclusive breastfeeding and/or formula until baby is six months old. However, it's important to note that not all babies are the same, and you should be aware of the thrust tongue reflex (especially if you plan to introduce real foods earlier than six months). The thrust tongue reflex is when any foreign substance is placed on baby's tongue, the tongue automatically projects (or thrusts) outward rather than back towards the esophagus.[3] If this happens when trying real foods, it's a sure sign that baby isn't ready yet. How cool is Mother Nature?! One should not forget all of the amazing survival instincts we are born with.

The other guidance I followed was starting Jack with a food that wasn't a fruit, so he wouldn't turn his nose up to any subsequent food introduced that wasn't sweet. Babies are naturally drawn to sweet foods, so the more sweetness they get, the less interested they are in low-sugar veggies, etc.[4]

Ironically, I thought I WAS doing baby-led weaning (BLW), although unaware there was a term for it, by not cutting Jack off from nursing before he was ready. Come to learn, that's not quite what baby-led weaning means. The term was invented by a nurse in the United Kingdom. In the UK, weaning means starting your baby on solid food.[5] It has nothing to do with ending breastfeeding, as it does in the United States. Don't you love it? Two countries who speak English yet have no idea what each other is saying. Not only when the Brits speak do they sound fancier than us Americans, but they have cooler terms for all of our words. Had an American been asked to coin this concept, we would have probably come up with something like "baby self feeds with hands". No mystery, no cute three-letter acronym. So boring.

It turns out, baby-led weaning is when you give your baby food in its original form (i.e. no purées), commonly cut into the shape of a stick so they can hold it, gnaw on it, or bite it if they have teeth. You also feed them whatever you're eating, just cut it up into the appropriate shape and size (about the size of your pinky finger). Additionally, each party has a role to play: Parents decide what to eat, when to eat, and where to eat, and baby decides whether to eat and how much to eat.[6]

If you're reacting like I did, you're gasping and saying, "I can't possibly do that. She'll choke!" Let's talk for a minute about the difference between choking and gagging and get educated on the gag reflex. The gag reflex is strong during the early months (remember the tongue thrust reflex) but shifts further back in the mouth and becomes similar to that of an adult around nine months of age. It's simply baby's body's way of saying, "Nah, not now. We're not prepared to swallow that yet," so that baby can basically reject any food he's not ready for and either chew it some more or spit it out. The other distinction between gagging and choking is gagging is usually accompanied by a coughing or fetching sound, and choking is silent. Choking is when a piece of food gets stuck in the airway and the baby is unable to breathe.[7] If a baby is coughing roughly or crying hard, then the airway is not fully blocked, and coughing and crying can actually help push it out.[8]

Once oriented with gagging versus choking, understanding how to present the food is another concept of baby-led weaning. There are two hand gestures referenced when it comes to baby-led weaning: the palmar grasp and the pincer grasp. The palmar grasp is what your baby will start out with around six months, and that's holding the food in a closed fist, literally in their palm. Hence, the stick-like shape for the foods at this age. Keep in mind that the food needs to be longer than fist-length because your baby will only be able to eat what's sticking out[9]; he doesn't understand how to access the food enclosed in his palm. If he can't see it, it pretty much doesn't exist in his mind. During the palmar phase, a neat idea for the slippery, hard to grasp foods, like bananas or mangos, is to roll the pieces in dry cereal crumbs (I actually opted for dry baby oatmeal).

A few months later, he will graduate from the palmar grasp to the pincer grasp, and this is the ability to pick up food with his pointer finger and thumb.[10] Think of some proper old lady eating dainty finger foods. Your baby will look like British royalty at afternoon tea, picking up chickpeas, blueberries, or Cheerios...pinky out.

One nugget of information I received from my pediatrician and tucked away was that until nine months old, introducing foods is more about getting them used to the concept of eating and the different flavors and textures than it is about caloric intake. Don't fall for the "food before one is just for fun" slogan that's floating around out there though. Babies do need the nutrition from real foods to complement their breastmilk/formula. Iron is one of these key nutrients, and it is low in breastmilk. That's okay since babies are born with four to six months of iron stored in their bodies.[11] Can we get a round of applause for Mother Nature again please? After that point, ensuring baby is getting exposed to appropriate sources of iron is important.

It's sometimes encouraged to do solid food feedings after a nursing or formula session when the baby isn't starving.[12] If you feed a starving baby, the baby may be frustrated with solids. It feels counterintuitive, but if you feed baby when he's not famished, he'll be more interested and curious. It's similar to not going grocery shopping when hungry. Sometimes I secretly love when I do that, though, because I end up with all these fun snacks in my house I would have never bought otherwise.

It's also around that nine-month mark that it is time to conduct the slew of "hold your breath and hope you're not feeding your baby poison" allergy and sensitivity tests. This includes peanuts, shellfish, soy, tree nuts, wheat, eggs, and dairy.[13] I also added strawberries to the list, although my pediatrician informed me that many of the reactions were really more to the pesticides than to the fruit itself. Therefore, to err on the side of caution I bought organic. In the past, doctors would advise parents to hold off or sometimes avoid altogether these common allergen foods, but the current guidance is to introduce them sooner rather than later for early detection and possible prevention.[14] Somewhere during Jack's ninth month, we started to run through this gamut of trickery treats.

A food allergy is basically the body's immune system misreading the food as a threat and reacting (hence the term, allergic reaction).[15] A food sensitivity (sometimes referred to as a food intolerance) is the body's digestive system not being able to process the food.[16] Both can make their presence known in many ways, some mild such as a rash and some severe such as trouble breathing. You are not a doctor, and now isn't the time to play one. If you notice any signs, contact your pediatrician. I erred on the side of caution and introduced these foods three days in a row, with all other foods consumed during those days foods Jack was previously exposed to in order to control the experiment. However, when it comes to this space, you should consult with your pediatrician on the best course of action for you, especially if there is a history of food allergies in your family.

Personally, I don't consume dairy (although I did expose him to it sufficiently to rule out any serious allergies or sensitivities). While this book is not intended to be about my dietary beliefs, I clearly have a hard time keeping my opinion to myself. I'll refrain from climbing on my soap box, but suffice it to say my stance is: Because I'm not a baby cow, I believe it was never intended for me to drink the milk of a cow. There is so much evidence supporting this logical thinking, and the one fun fact I must share with you is that as humans, about 75% of us lose the gene to break down lactose after weaning, and for many the ability to break it down post-weaning is at about 10–15% what it was when first born. This is why lactose intolerance, i.e. what happens when the body lacks the enzymes needed to break down lactose, a natural sugar found in milk, is so common.[17] Additionally, dairy can be constipating for babies.[18] If you practice extended breastfeeding, there really is no reason to ever give your baby whole milk.

Two other ingredients to be mindful of during the introduction of real foods are salt and refined sugar. In theory, both should be limited or altogether avoided. Here's the deal: You should limit sodium intake for 6- to 12-month-olds to 370 mg per day, according to the National Academics of Science Engineering and Medicine because baby's tiny kidneys can only handle so much.[19] Even if you're heavy on the saltshaker for yourself, keep it bland for baby.

Limiting sugar, on the other hand, is more about giving baby the chance to acquire tastes for flavors other than sweet.[20] As mentioned previously, babies are naturally drawn to sweet things. Again, this isn't a diet book, but unless you live under a rock, you should be well aware of the downsides to a sugary diet at any age. If despite all the evidence, you're someone with a sweet tooth and you plan to always have sweets around your house and available to your children, then you do you. But perhaps, maybe we could also view this as a time to clean up our own diets so that we can feel our best for baby and set a good example?

A Note on Honey

Infant botulism is serious because the bacteria is toxic and unable to be processed by baby's digestive system under age one.[21] Since we have enough on our plates (see what I did there) as new moms, regardless on where you stand on sugar, let's just tell honey to buzz off until baby has completed his first trip around the sun.

What Worked for Me

Fascinated and still a little confused, I decided to give baby-led weaning a test drive with some pasta. Overall, I wouldn't say baby-led weaning was a slam dunk for us, but it was definitely more successful than the purées.

I'm not going to lie, baby-led weaning was pretty stressful at times. Having not been programed to give whole food to a baby this young, I had to rewire my brain to not think he's going to choke all the time. Understanding the difference between choking and gagging and knowing about the gag reflex helped, and it's something I wish I researched sooner than I did. It would have saved me from the several times I fish-hooked food out of his mouth, panicking that it was going to get lodged in his throat.

I confused gagging with choking more often than not, and while you should NEVER leave your baby unattended during mealtime (think of yourself as the Secret Service and your baby as the POTUS), it is more relaxing when you are aware of the gag reflex.

Thankfully I never had a choking experience with Jack, but I'm going to pull a "do as I say not as I do" moment: Get CPR certified. I had full intentions of taking a course with Justin, but the course at the hospital kept filling up every month by the time I remembered to register. Then all hell broke loose with COVID-19, and hospital classes were a thing of the past. I kick myself for not doing it, and while I've read and watched videos online, I still wish I took the course. God-willing as mamas we never have to use it, but it'll give us confidence should the need unfortunately arise; we'll be prepared and less panicked.

In case you're wondering whether or not having teeth helps with baby-led weaning, I can tell you my experience. Jack popped teeth pretty early. At four months of age, he had his first two teeth, and he had a few more by the time we started eating. Let's be clear, though, he was pretty clueless as to what to do with them, and they didn't necessarily benefit us in any way for feedings. Even though you're giving your baby food in its original form, they're gumming the food to mash it up, not using their front chompers.

Regarding the allergy "tests", I never got around to shellfish. Truth is, we never eat it, so it was just an inconvenience to go out of my way to get shellfish for my baby to try when he'd probably never be offered it again until he was older. Not my proudest rebel moment, but I'm not going to act like I followed the rules to a T when I didn't entirely. I'm happy to report that for the other common offenders, we had no issues. To this day, peanut butter is still hands down Jack's favorite food.

What we need to have at mealtime is monk-like patience. In the heat of a "he's denying everything I give him" moment, we panic and fear that baby will never eat anything and will look like a skeleton and wither away, but that is so unlikely.

You know that phrase "acquired taste"? That term applies to almost every food I introduced to Jack. Learn from me: Don't give up! Not every food (in fact, no other food) was love at first sight like peanut butter was. Even if a food is ignored or spit out weeks and weeks in a row, sometimes a baby needs to be exposed to a food many times before willing to accept. I distinctly remember this happening with broccoli and peas, two green foods I serve often. After meal upon meal of poo-pooing these foods, something just clicked. One night Jack started shoving peas into his mouth like he was Lucy and Ethel working at the chocolate factory conveyor belt. However, just because baby loved a food one day, he may turn his nose up at it the next day and then treat it like a long-lost friend the day after. It can be a fickle relationship for sure.

While I missed so many of my favorite restaurants and hoped every day that they would survive the storm of the pandemic, I consider myself lucky to have avoided bringing Jack out to eat on a regular basis due to restrictions. When I did take him out before the outbreak of COVID-19, it was not relaxing at all unless he was asleep in the stroller. Babies, it turns out, are not meant to sit at the table for an hour plus, and especially not for the part between the menus being taken away and the food being served. This all screamed BORING to my little guy who wasn't interested in sipping cocktails or small talk.

Whether you're spoon feeding or baby-led weaning, neither are all that convenient when you're out, albeit baby-led weaning is slightly easier. However, the choking fear rises to a new level because now you're not home. There are people watching you, and you didn't cook nor prep the food your baby is eating. And the catch-22 is you'd like a second glass of wine to take the edge off before the first one has even hit your belly, but you can't because you're breastfeeding, nor can you afford for your senses to be dulled in case you have to react at the speed of light and save your baby from choking. Somehow your husband is oblivious to all of this, happily drinking a beer and eating his burger, and you're contemplating what you ever saw in him anyway.

If on the other hand you have one of those angelic babies who just sits in their highchair and happily plays with the menu the entire meal, I applaud you, Mama. Chances are you did nothing to deserve that round of applause and that's just how your baby is wired, but I applaud you, nevertheless. If you have a baby who is more like mine, treating the water glasses like a splash park and requesting a full tour of the restaurant for the tenth time, completely distraught that you're not tall enough to lift him up so he can touch the red exit sign over every door, it's okay to just stay home. Or get takeout. Or eat a bag of microwave popcorn for dinner in silent solitude after you've finally wrestled your alligator to bed.

I didn't just avoid meals out, I avoided meals with people, period, thanks to social distancing. Yes, it was lonely at times, but I didn't have the noise of busybody nosy people who think offering my baby chocolate after dinner (which is inconveniently an hour before bedtime) is a good idea. I was able, without judgement, to feed my baby in a way that I felt would give him the best nutrition.

I was forced (but it felt more like I was privileged) to prepare and eat meals at home, just the three of us, and it was a huge relief because the meal itself could be stressful enough. In reality, mealtime etiquette training does not need to (and should not) begin at the same time you introduce solids. Rebelling against eating out and long meals does not mean your baby is going to turn out to be the most ill-mannered dinner guest, belching and refusing the food in front of him. The reality is that a meal with a baby is at most fifteen minutes, and it is actually impossible to teach manners to a baby this young. Their brains aren't even close to being able to understand such sophisticated concepts as to which fork is the salad fork and to keep elbows off the table.

One of the rare moments of brilliance I had when creating our baby registry was the highchair selection. I remember looking at the highchairs in the store, marveling how all of them had cloth seat covers. So many seams and cracks. They looked like they were just begging for food stains and hidden crumbs. Sure, you could take the fabric cushions off and put them in the washing machine, but doing that on a daily basis felt like a laborious task. Moms do not need to add any more unnecessary labor to their days! I declined adding one to my registry from the store and instead found one online that had a leather seat (easy to wipe down) and a removable table-top tray for washing.

I'm glad I had that lightbulb moment because baby-led weaning can get pretty messy. We're talking Pablo Picasso style at every meal. Then, there is the floor. If your highchair is over carpet, you need to rip that up immediately, or find another spot in the house that is hard flooring for mealtime. Proportionately speaking, the size of a highchair tray compared to the amount of food served to a baby is easily a 10:1 ratio, meaning the food only takes up a tenth of the tray, and there should be more than enough space for the food. It sounds logical in theory, but when Jack realized he could send that food flying over the side of the highchair, he'd squeal in delight and send peanut butter toast pieces, pasta, and blueberries as far as he could. His grand finale, which was both impressive and cringeworthy to watch, was the "I'm all done with this meal...time to clear my plate" act, in which he'd turn his right arm into the equivalent of a windshield wiper on the highest setting during a monsoon and swipe the tray back and forth at lightning speed until everything had been shot on the floor.

On a good night, we maybe got five minutes with Jack in his highchair while he explored what I'd put in front of him. On a bad night, he demanded to be let out immediately. He would then contently sit on one of our laps, exploring and experimenting with our utensils and the foods on our plates, oftentimes with the intent focus of an OR surgeon.

I know there are many who, if they watched me parent, would be horrified, and dinnertime is no exception. Not only does he sleep in my bed and was breastfed past one year of age, I've also "allowed" the "bad habit" of him sitting with us at the table. How will I ever break him of this, my spoiled little brat?!

Purées are not his thing. Highchair seats, or anything that straps him in (including car seats and strollers), make him incredibly unhappy. Parents who listen to his needs and respond accordingly, even if the response is totally unconventional? Now, that's his jam.

It is our job as parents to tune into our baby and understand their needs. If we don't do this, and instead follow some one-size-fits-all parenting manual, not only are we missing the mark and making our lives more difficult than they need to be, but we're also not creating the secure, trusting relationship with our baby that is SO CRITICAL to their maturity and development.

I forewent bottle feeding once I was permanently quarantined at home. I also let him decide how much he wanted to eat and stopped forcing purées in his mouth every day (it was painful to throw away my hard work). I tried a mix of mush and solids to see what interested him and what didn't. And, there were days he consumed nothing but breast milk and potato chips.

What was important was that he was a healthy weight and height and physically and mentally progressing properly. We live in a food-centric culture and tend to overemphasize the importance of a balanced diet (ironic because the obesity rate has never been higher). While I'm not saying potato chips are a proper meal, it is most definitely not the end of the world if they end up on the menu here and there.

From the time we started feeding Jack solids to the time he was fisting pasta into his mouth like a college kid who just smoked marijuana for the first time was actually only a few short months. Be patient (challenge your inner Buddhist monk), be consistent, and be as healthy as possible without driving yourself crazy. Avoid salt, avoid sugar (you know where I stand here), and offer a variety of foods. Eventually some will stick, some will come with time, and some he may never enjoy.

7

Separation Anxiety
Child Care

ROAD TO REBELLION

I was raised by a stay-at-home mom. I never went to daycare nor summer camp. I'd say that's probably why I'm as introverted and hermit-like as I am, but my sister was raised in the same household and she's a social butterfly. Nevertheless, I felt strongly about the importance of one-on-one attention in the early years. This was before I did any research. This was just pure gut talking. Remember—instinct versus instruction. Unfortunately, I also felt strongly about being able to afford our mortgage payment and utility bills, so quitting my job was not an option. I knew I had to come up with a solution that didn't involve dropping my four-month-old baby off at a daycare center with dozens of other children for ten hours per day, five days per week. I get a knot in my stomach just thinking about it.

I say four-month-old because that's about how long I'd be home with my baby before my maternity leave was over and I had to return to work. I originally considered myself fortunate that I had a sixteen-week, paid maternity leave at my company.

It wasn't until talking to some of my European colleagues that I started to realize maybe I wasn't as fortunate as I originally thought. At the time, I was working on a big global project, and many of my non-U.S. coworkers would often ask me how long I'd be out from work. When I told them roughly sixteen weeks from when the baby was born, they were shocked. So many of them had months (some even over a year) of time off with their newborns, and much of that time was full or partially paid!

Meanwhile, I was answering work emails in the delivery room from my cell phone. My own doing, I know, but no one at my job was telling me to stand down. The reality is they were squeezing every last minute out of me that they could.

Knowing there wasn't much I could do to change the maternity leave policy in less than nine months, I knew I had to come up with a game plan for when I went back to work. At the time, the plan I crafted felt like a genius plan, and I'm SO GRATEFUL I was naïve and ignorant, or I would have never seen this plan through. Suffice it to say it wasn't my most brilliant thought bubble: I asked my dad to watch the baby.

Allow me to draw your attention back to the beginning of this chapter. I said I was raised by a stay-at-home mom, not a stay-at-home dad. In fact, my dad wasn't home often at all, being the sole income provider for our family. Yet here I was, asking him to watch the baby when I wasn't even sure if he ever changed a diaper. What was I thinking?! Oh, my friends, I'll say it again, you are so beautifully ignorant before you have a baby. I just figured it couldn't be that hard: feed the baby, change the baby, and make sure the baby takes naps. I was hoping if he could get me through the first year or so, I'd reassess childcare then. At least the baby would be at our house and getting one-on-one attention with a loving family member. In addition, we were more than willing to compensate him. It wasn't about the cost; we were fortunate enough to be able to afford the price of traditional day care, I just didn't want Jack to leave the house or be with a stranger.

As luck would have it, my dad was conveniently finding himself with extra time on his hands just over one week after Jack was due to arrive. At age sixty-one, he had an awful lot of energy that my mom felt needed to be channeled, or he surely would drive her insane. So as my belly grew, I asked him if he would watch the baby for me while I was at work. He was dumbfounded (and probably wondering if I was just plain dumb). In the moment, it felt logical. I had other friends whose retired grandparent(s) watched the babies, and their kids were kept alive. I had grandiose plans for how he would spend the days with Jack. I even made him learn sign language before Jack was born because I read it was a great thing to teach babies before they can talk.

My confidence grew even more when around ten weeks postpartum, my parents watched Jack for us one night so we could go out to dinner—our first official date night as parents. It went swimmingly. I left them with pages of instructions, and Jack was an angel. He even drank a bottle before bed and went to sleep and stayed asleep the whole time we were gone. Therefore, I had false confidence that Jack would be a breeze during the day, if he had let someone else put him to sleep at night.

The reality, though, was that my dad was so unfit for the job it was comical. I say that tongue in cheek and with love in my heart because he was actually a really good dad when I was growing up. (Truth is my mom has always been my favorite parent, by a landslide. So, I feel relatively objective in stating he was a good dad, albeit I am his daughter.) He was fun, funny, and loving. He made us a priority, and I have countless memories of good times with him while I was growing up. I just forgot babies don't have conscious memories, so I actually had absolutely no personal recommendation for my dad as a caregiver. These "countless memories" were from about the age of four and older, which was probably the age I was when my mom let my dad do things with us solo.

My dad wanted to be called Pops by his grandkids, so from Jack's birthdate onward, he was no longer Dad and always Pops. In the few weeks leading up to my return to work (quite possibly the most depressing few weeks of my entire existence), I started "training" him. I gave him written instructions, I had him practice feeding Jack the bottle, and I had him practice putting him down for naps. I gave him a printout of our daily routine, which consisted of outdoor walks, reading books, and play time. I had him observe me so he would be able to imitate my demeanor when flying solo. After several weeks of nanny bootcamp, he officially became Nanny Pops.

In those preceding weeks, I told myself every day it would be fine. This was normal; everyone was sad before they went back to work, but I had to do it. Every working mom does it, and so can I. It's only ten hours per day if you include the commute time, and I had Fridays either off or I would be working from home.

In the end, none of the self-talk helped. I had a pit in my stomach, and I cried the entire day the day before I went back into the office. While doing our daily reading, I could not finish *The Wonderful Things You Will Be* children's book because I was sobbing so hard. Jack, being the gentleman that he is, didn't draw any attention to the tears streaming down my face.

Working from the office was just as horrible as I had imagined, even though I loved my job. Before Jack, I was definitely guilty of being a workaholic. I loved the culture in my company, I loved the challenge of the work I did, and I enjoyed continued success and promotion. So, it's not like I went back to some job I despised or a boss that I hated. Quite the opposite, in fact.

Yet, the first couple of months were awful. There's no sugar coating it. Nanny Pops was all sorts of wrong for Jack. He wasn't soft (He doesn't talk, he bellows.), he wasn't calming (He oozes anxiety.), and worst of all (from Jack's point of view) he wasn't me. Jack would fight him for naps, refuse to drink from his bottle, and rarely crack a smile when they were alone.

One of the biggest issues Nanny Pops was having was getting Jack to settle for a nap. I consciously (and regrettably, in retrospect) rarely put Jack to sleep for naps by nursing him when I was on maternity leave because I knew that wasn't something Nanny Pops would be able to do. (Although we often joked about buying him one of those hilarious contraptions that Robert DeNiro had in *Meet the Fockers*). Instead, I usually rocked him and played the same soundtrack of lullabies as a sleep queue. Nanny Pops was well-trained on this, but it didn't matter how he did it. Jack would have a screaming meltdown every time he tried. For whatever bizarre reason, Nanny Pops would resort to walking him around outside to settle him down.

I think he did it because he didn't want to hear him screaming in the house, and somehow the fresh air calmed them both down; but that was the only way he could get him to fall asleep. I'd have been fine with this solution if it was summertime, but in late November and early December in the Northeast, I now added "pneumonia" to my list of concerns over Jack being with Nanny Pops all day.

I missed Jack tremendously. I stressed constantly about whether he was unhappy with Nanny Pops (which 99% of the time I'm sure he was) or whether Nanny Pops was feeling overwhelmed (which 99% of the time he probably was). I was managing to make it through my workload and pull myself together enough to seem like someone who knew what she was talking about, but I knew it wasn't sustainable.

I used to lie awake in the middle of the night (oftentimes while nursing), thinking about how I could be home more or what expenses we could cut so I could quit and we could survive on one salary. Then, I'd spend other sleepless nights racking my brain for how I could find a different caregiver Jack would like more and who I would feel was more qualified. (At this point in the journey, I think Elmo would have met both of those requirements.) Thoughts I'd never thought I'd have kept me up all night. I had many girlfriends who were all like, "I was so ready to come back to work," when their maternity leave was over, so I just assumed I'd feel the same way, since I did enjoy my job.

Redefining Normal

In the United States, sixteen weeks paid leave is considered a generous maternity leave benefit. Some women have as little as six weeks off. In fact, the United States is the only developed country in the world that does not mandate paid leave for new mothers.[1] Disgusting, isn't it? It should be illegal for a mother to be separated from her baby at six weeks of age. It should be illegal to expect a new mom to be able to function like a working adult just six weeks after giving birth.

On the other end of the spectrum, Hungary allows mothers up to three years of paid time off for each child.[2] I know you can't schedule a pregnancy like you can a doctor's appointment or a dinner reservation, but if you're able to have children consecutively only a few years apart, you could have upwards of six years off. It gets better! Italy and the Netherlands actually require mandatory time off weeks BEFORE the baby actually arrives, not just after.[3] What a novel concept, give the soon-to-be mama some time to rest and prepare, eliminating any stress from work.

The system in the U.S. is not supporting mothers, and it's incredibly frustrating and disheartening. A 2011 report published by the U.S. Census Bureau showed that only 22% of women did not return to work after having a baby, down from 36% in the early 1980s.[4] The reality is, it's not getting any cheaper to live. I know I joked about not being able to afford my mortgage earlier, but it's true. The number of dual income households now is higher than it's ever been.[5] Families are put in a difficult position, oftentimes with their hearts and their bills in direct conflict. They want to practice attachment parenting, but they can't afford to stay away from the office.

Mamas, you're not crazy if when you listen to your inner voice and not all of the outside influences, it feels "off" when you're apart from your baby. I don't mean because you have mom guilt from being away from her, I mean literally you feel out of balance. Guess why? Because for the first several years of life, mother and baby are meant to be one unit![6] Just because you evicted that little nugget from your uterus after ten months doesn't mean you aren't supposed to continue to live in harmony.

There is a theory that because children under the age of three have little concept of duration of time, they have a hard time understanding if mama isn't available NOW, mama is never going to be available (even if all mama did was try to go to the bathroom in peace and quiet). Once a child hits age three or so, they understand that a few minutes is different from a few days, etc., and separation becomes easier for both child and mama.[7]

I digress, but my point is, the way I was feeling was okay even though I kept thinking I must just be overreacting or being a first-time over-the-top mom. (I've been accused of being over the top once or twice before.)

Please, don't walk away from this section thinking I'm promoting new moms to rebel against daycare, put their asses on the line, and play hooky from their jobs. But, stopping and questioning the social norm and evaluating your situation so that you are comfortable with where your baby is and who your baby is with is completely acceptable.

I have coworkers who during COVID-19 were doing happy dances when their daycares reopened. It does work for some! My point is we do NOT have to feel cornered into returning to work full time and putting our baby in daycare. Explore options like temporarily switching to part-time or take a longer, unpaid leave.

You can bet your ass, however, that I'm promoting rebelling against some government-dictated duration where you're told how long you are allowed to be home with your child. Tune in to your inner self; she knows how long she needs to be with her baby.

Listen, I know some women who went back to work EARLY because their postpartum depression was so bad, and they needed some sense of normalcy. So, I'm not saying every mama is meant to strap her baby to her chest and stay together around the clock for a year, but I know far too many women who were fraught with sorrow over having to go back to work and to be separated from their baby at six weeks, eight weeks, twelve weeks, etc. Countless mamas who agonize over returning to work eventually settle into a new norm of long periods of separation. The few mamas I do know who decided not to return to work (or went back to work only for a few weeks and then quit) said it's the best decision they've ever made.

Let's band together and commit to having the uncomfortable conversations with our spouses or bosses about different options, where we may bring home less pay, because we can't discount the price of the emotional trauma we may be incurring by sticking to our pre-baby job. An uncomfortable conversation or two is nothing in comparison to the discomfort we might feel every day we leave the house for work.

It's not a forever decision, it's a temporary change. This does not mean we're throwing our careers away. I know women who have made a career change once their children were old enough. I have a friend who didn't go back to work for eight months because that's how long it took her daughter to start drinking from the bottle, but she did in fact go back! This is like anything else in life. If you have the drive, you'll find a way. Settling for less than ideal doesn't have to be our only option. We only get one shot at these early years, and before we know it they'll be putting on their backpacks for school.

A fellow mama told me now that she's passed the pre-K years, she wishes she took more time to be home. The years are so short in retrospect.

Who cares about what you previously thought you were supposed to do with regards to work? Now that you have this little precious ball of life and you are the apple of her eye, you're allowed to change your mind. You're allowed to question your prior thinking. You're allowed to make some lifestyle changes so that you can maximize your time cultivating your relationship with your baby.

WHAT WORKED FOR ME

I couldn't do it. To this day I tell my husband I would have quit my job before leaving Jack in a daycare, and that's not because I think they're all run by the lady who ran Mathilda's orphanage.

Most of these daycare centers are run by caring, loving individuals, but there is an actual biological need for a baby to be with his or her mom. It's not made up. What worries me is the impact of today's households, which have the highest number of dual incomes, resorting to placing their newborns in childcare. In my humble opinion, we're by far the most twisted generation. This is the result of many factors, including the garbage food we eat and the social media we scroll, but lack of time with parents at such an early age must be an impacting factor.

While feeling confident in my decision to not put Jack in daycare, I was feeling unsure about my decision to have my non-maternal father watching Jack.

I had been back to work for two months when the new year came. I always make News Year's resolutions. (Ain't nothing wrong with being basic every now and again; I also get a pumpkin spiced latté in September every year too.) One of my resolutions was to work from home fifty percent of the time. I was having a hard time being apart from Jack, in case that isn't blatantly obvious to you by now. I went back to work the first of November, so I took time off around Thanksgiving and Christmas and came home early at least one or two days per week. I was working from home often, but it never felt like enough. The resolution was mostly because I missed Jack greatly, but I also wanted to supervise the babysitter.

I did a good job sticking to my New Year's resolution in January and February. Being home more often allowed me to be more available for feedings and to put Jack down for naps. When I was in the office, he would literally drink a total of one ounce from the bottle throughout the day until I came home.

Then, in early March, I took a week off to celebrate my wedding anniversary (with Jack in tow) in Vermont. It was that week the coronavirus became real in the United States. I remember things started heating up Wednesday of that week, and I decided I'd make sure when I returned to work on Monday, I'd bring home much of my office supplies. Two days later, grocery stores were out of toilet paper and flour, and I had received an email from work saying not to come into the office for two weeks.

The pandemic changed my life in many ways, but it also saved my career and my sanity. It transformed me into a stay-at-home working mom...a "have your cake and eat it too" moment. I changed the way I worked, and it worked.

Nanny Pops would still come to watch Jack Monday through Thursday (with the exception of certain weeks where my COVID-19 paranoia was at an all-time high). I would take necessary work meetings during the day, but I maximized all of Jack's awake time with him. I worked when he napped, and then I'd save the rest of my work for when he went to bed. (The transition from two naps to one nap was such a kick in the crotch.) I'd prop myself up in bed next to him, laptop lighting up the otherwise pitch-black room, and I'd pound away on the keyboard until I was caught up for the day.

It was life-altering for all of us: Justin and me as parents, my dad as a caregiver, and Jack as a developing baby. Within a month I had pretty much retired my breast pump, for the first time truly embracing the concept of "nursing on demand" which I wish I did from the beginning. Instead, I was always stressing about getting him on a schedule so that it would be easier when I was in the office. Quite honestly, I think we all took a huge sigh of relief that the HBIC was home. Nanny Pops became more of a helper than the sole caregiver. Rarely did he have more than an hour or so alone with Jack before either Justin or I took a break from work for a visit. Jack was more at ease, knowing I was home and having almost constant access to me. And Justin, well, I think he was grateful to stop receiving "please get your ass home I'm worried Jack is upset" text messages every time he left the house to see a client.

If you are assuming that my performance at work likely suffered as a result, which is what led to writing this book to supplement my income, it was quite the opposite! I was much more relaxed about things at home, allowing me to focus on my work. I was even awarded one of the few MVP awards at the end of the big project we were working on. My career was flourishing, and I was doing it all in yoga pants with a baby latched to my nipple.

Something else magical happened while we were quarantining. I can't pinpoint the exact moment, but somewhere amongst the madness, Jack went from barely tolerating my dad, to being obsessed with him. "Best friends" is only one of many phrases to describe what their relationship transformed into. As Jack got older and could walk and talk, he'd stand by the front window and ask, "Pops?" any time my dad wasn't at the house (Speaking of talking, life was such a shitshow for my dad and Jack that they never got around to using sign language). When Pops did arrive, Jack would visibly shake with excitement at the sight of him. Make no mistake, I was still this boy's favorite human by a landslide, but we made strides in a matter of months with Nanny Pops.

I'm not sure how things would have looked if COVID-19 never happened. Would my work from home fifty percent of the time resolution have been enough? Would I even have been able to realistically swing it? How would I have handled the first time I had to travel for work (which given the job I had, would have been inevitable at some point)? Would I have totally rebelled and quit?

Those questions are of course rhetorical, but regardless, I am forever grateful and eternally indebted to Nanny Pops for toughing it out during those early months, for loving Jack and not giving up on us, and for listening (mostly) to my never-ending list of rules.

8

Guilty as Charged
Mom Guilt

ROAD TO REBELLION

These topics I've discussed and decisions I've made hopefully have not implied that motherhood has been a walk in the park for me. Au contraire, my friend. Some days it's like walking across hot coals. Whether you had an epidural or you labored au naturale, whether you feed with bottle or breast, whether you're cribbing it or co-sleeping, we ALL face similar mama challenges—and mom guilt is at the TOP of the list.

Much to my surprise, upon consulting Merriam-Webster online for the term "mom guilt", I was informed, "The word you've entered isn't in the dictionary." Forced to take matters into my own hands, I've defined this internal monster as "the soul sucking, crippling sensation that you're not doing enough, and most definitely completely ruining your child's entire life." Sound familiar?

I was a stickler for safety. Mobile babies are constantly cruising for a bruising, and for eleven months I was successful in keeping Jack out of harm's way...minus that one time when he was nine weeks old and I clipped his fingertip with the nail clippers. Why don't babies came with nails that don't grow for the first twelve months? And, what a total shrew I was to my husband and my dad sometimes, berating them to be more careful, "don't hold him like that, you're not close enough to him, he's going to get hurt", etc. I can just hear my nagging voice. I was incredibly careful, and he rarely got hurt on my watch. Yes, Jack would bang into things sometimes, usually when he was learning to crawl and stand up, but nothing major.

Until one inconspicuous Monday, I decided I would take him out for a walk on my lunch break. It was a beautiful day. After we finished eating, I put on my sneakers and sunglasses, put a sun bonnet on Jack, and we walked out the front door like I would do any of the other countless times we've gone for a stroll. Justin was going to meet us at the garage so he could get the stroller (the benefits of quarantining…family walks at lunch time). As I was talking to Justin about something that I can't recall, I walked down the first step of our front patio to the driveway and tripped OVER NOTHING. I just lost my footing on the step down, my ankle twisted, and I fell to the ground with Jack in my arms. On…the… pavement.

Some deep subconscious maternal instinct kicked in. I didn't let go of him until we were about six inches from the ground, at which point I had to do something or we were both going to slam our heads on the driveway. Mind you, I don't have any conscious memory of this; this is all from my husband's eyewitness account. I had released my tight grip on him to put out my arms, and my perfect baby boy hit his head on the driveway and screamed.

Completely ignoring the pain in my ankle, I scooped him into my arms and held him so close, shushing him and feeling on his head for a bump. I felt nothing but sheer panic that I may have permanently damaged Jack. It was a quick search; my hand was immediately greeted by an egg-sized bump on the top of the back of his head, and my heart sank.

The proceeding set of events were a bit of a whirlwind, but it went something like this: Justin calling the pediatrician, the pediatrician telling us to go to urgent care, my dad telling us he's fine it's just a bump, and my ankle swelling to the size of a balloon.

The next thing I knew I was in urgent care, in the middle of a goddamn pandemic, wearing a face mask with my baby in my arms. It wasn't even thirty minutes after the incident, and Jack was pointing and oohing obsessively at the lit up red exit sign in the waiting room, oblivious to the bump on his head. Anyone who saw us would assume we were there because I twisted my ankle and my baby was just along for the ride. Jack was totally over the incident, and I was completely distraught and beside myself with anxiety, stress, and guilt. We had a CT scan done just to be on the safe side, and the scan showed that there was no damage, just a bump that would go away in a couple of days. Still to this day I can't talk about placing my tiny eleven-month-old baby in that giant machine and holding him while they did the scan...Jack looking up at me scared and confused as to where we were and what was going on.

The bump was gone within forty-eight hours. I beat myself up far longer than that. I couldn't get over it. I couldn't stop replaying it in my head, torturing myself with the memory. I kept thinking how I wouldn't be able to live with myself if it resulted in something bad happening to him. The worst part of it all was that I did nothing wrong! My shoes were tied, I wasn't distracted, it was a beautiful sunny day—no rain, snow, or ice to blame it on. I agonized over it, continually playing the "what if" game. What if I just didn't decide to take a walk that day or what if I went out through the garage instead of the front door? What if I had Justin carry him instead? All the scenarios of preventing the fall played in my head. My mom guilt was through the roof. I overcompensated during the following weeks by barely leaving his side, worried he'd either get hurt again or have a delayed reaction to the head trauma.

Let me pause here and tell you that I enjoy my son thoroughly, and being connected at the hip with him is not exactly my idea of a burden. The older he gets and the more we can interact and dialogue, the more and more I fall in love with him, which I didn't think was possible considering my heart has been on the verge of bursting since day one. I remember talking with some work girlfriends during the few months I was actually in the office, and I commented on how I never get sick of him and I could be with him 24/7. They laughed and said, "Oh, that's because he's only six months old." I just smiled, but inside I thought, "Will I really get sick of my baby?" Months later, I still felt the same way. We have such a bond, and everything feels right when I with him. I can't exactly explain it but know that I enjoy my time with him; and I'm with him as often as I am because I want to be, not because I feel guilty otherwise.

But, sometimes being connected at the hip does not allow for many (or any) of mama's chores to get done, or her own needs to get met, which can lead to feeling extra guilty—guilty for leaving my son to do some laundry or cooking and guilty that I haven't done laundry or cooked (or probably showered) in what feels like ten years.

The term "attachment parenting" always created a literal image in my mind—a mom, wearing her baby in one of those baby carriers, which pre-pregnancy I never saw myself doing. I assumed I would just hold my baby, and I did hold him a lot; however, even ten pounds can start to feel like 100 after a while and is not comfortable for long durations.

I did, of course, register for two baby carriers because, again, why not? One was bulky and looked and felt like a hiking backpack. The other was chic and simple, like a bathing suit sarong wrap. I assumed this is the one I'd wear most often, as the bulky one seemed impractical. Jack wanted to be connected (or as they say, attached) to me at all times. I decided when he was a few weeks old to try out the chic baby wrap with the help of my dad when he was over for a pre-nanny visit.

Attempting to put this thing on felt like we were playing a life-size game of cat's cradle, my limbs were fingers and the wrap the string. It was impossible, and every variation we tried seemed to have a hole Jack would be able to slide through. It was just as challenging to get it off me as it was to get it on me, and I ended up returning it shortly after. I went back to the old-fashioned isometric bicep curl position, and when Jack was a little older, I decided I'd try the "bulky" baby carrier.

Turns out that bulkiness is strategic, designed to give you maximum support as your baby grows bigger (because try as we might, we can't keep them little forever).

I was guilt-ridden about not keeping him safe enough, guilt-ridden about being apart from him, and if that's not enough, I was also guilt-ridden about any evils he might hear, see, or eat. (The three wise Japanese monkeys were mocking me, with their little hands covering their ears, eyes, and mouth in order to hear no evil, see no evil, speak no evil!)

Forgive me Father for I have sinned; it has been a shit-ton of time since my last confession, and these are my sins: I used the Lord's name in vain once or twice (okay, maybe more than that). I'll admit my mouth could benefit from being washed out with soap from time to time. While I'm far from a trucker, the F bomb slips, and some of the expressions I use could be considered by some as crude. I'm not particularly bothered by it, even though in an ideal world I'd clean it up. It's just never been a priority. The older Jack got, though, the more I started begrudgingly agreeing with my mom when she'd said things like, "You're going to really have to cut out the cuss words, Laura." It doesn't matter how old you are, when your mom tells you something that you know is right, even though you don't want to hear it, you find yourself having a difficult time admitting it. It can't just be me, right?

My son is a monster in the car. We drove four hours to Maine when he was just over a year old, and it felt like four days. I finally caved and pulled out my cell phone to play nursery rhyme videos on YouTube. He watched them for eleven minutes. That's less than five percent of our total car time. I could have allowed myself to feel bad about it, but for the love of all things sane, I was losing my goddamn mind and so was Jack. Justin probably was too, but that son of a gun was in the driver's seat, practically

SECRET WEAPONS

Ergobaby 360

Mamas, I've worn this so many times, and it is LIFE CHANGING. It's such a win that I'm tripping over my words to get them all on paper. You and baby will never be happier. Baby is as close to mommy as humanly possible, and mommy has BOTH HANDS free.

I've done laundry, gone for walks/hikes, cooked meals, taken a poop, all while wearing the Ergo. I remember Jack once took a two-and-a-half-hour nap in the Ergo. Yes, the same Jack who at that age would have probably slept a maximum of forty minutes in his Pack 'n Play at one time.

I cannot emphasize enough how much freedom and comfort this carrier gave me. While definitely a bit pricey (retailed at $150 at the time), it was absolutely worth the investment. Or, if you're lucky, register for one and it'll be gifted to you!

a world away from the hell I was living through in the backseat. Those eleven minutes were pure bliss, and I told the screen time mom guilt to take a hike.

I'm not a big TV girl myself. We don't have one in our bedroom, and even when Justin and I were dating, I couldn't sleep if he left his on to fall asleep to. Before Justin, I bought a fancy TV when I lived alone, and one of my best friends joked and said, "Well, that's a very expensive knickknack for you, wouldn't you say?" Today, we don't have cable (Does anyone under the age of sixty have cable?), but we have all the streaming apps. The TV is rarely on when Jack is awake, so incidentally it's not a focus for him.

As for the third monkey, I've modified him from "speak" to "eat". If you recall from chapter six, I harbored mom guilt far too long over Jack's ingestion of formula.

REDEFINING NORMAL

If you decide to be a rebel in only ONE area from this book, make it this one. But, please don't sell yourself short like that. Be a badass bitty and rebel in all the areas you want. Similar to the word "busy", "mom guilt" is another badge of honor in our dysfunctional society. However, it's not cool to be busy, and it's not cool to have mom guilt either. It's also REALLY bad for your mental health to let mom guilt get the best of you. Your baby loves you. It's incredible, I know, since we are so imperfect in our own eyes, but we're actually super perfect in our babies' eyes. I do understand how tempting it is to use it as an excuse to skip the office happy hour or the Zumba class your coworker keeps trying to drag you to: "Ugh, sorry, I just can't commit. I already feel so guilty for how little I've seen my baby this week." Let's come up with something better.

We're going to work through this together. Repeat after me: I'm not a terrible mom if my baby physically gets hurt, I'm not a terrible mom if I'm not with my baby around the clock, and I'm not a terrible mom if my baby is exposed to some evil of the world. The sooner you believe this, I swear your grey hairs will instantly slow down. (They're never going to stop, though. It's a byproduct of motherhood that you have to come to terms with.)

Shit happens. No one wants their baby to get hurt. If you do, you're some sort of sociopath, and you probably picked this book up in error. The majority of mamas would love to wrap their baby in bubble wrap from day one, only taking it off long enough to take some adorable photos of their perfect little doll. Needless to say, your baby getting hurt is one of the major reasons for mom guilt. How do we compensate? We hover. Like an annoying gnat, we're on top of our babies to make sure we prevent as many falls and slips as possible.

We're going to go insane if we keep this up, and as you saw from me, it isn't a guarantee to keep your baby free and clear! I'll tell you what else wasn't doing me any good: telling others about the accident. I would share the story of the incident, feeling so ashamed, yet these other parents would reply by telling me to not beat myself up. Then, they proceeded to tell an even worse story of their own! I heard stories about six-month-olds who fell off beds, toddlers who got electrocuted, and I shit you not, one girlfriend told me she was cutting her son's finger nails and one of the clippings flew into his eye...and she had to get it out with tweezers because she was afraid he'd go blind. (Yes, I was thinking the same thing—poking tweezers in his eye might make him go blind quicker than a fingernail clipping.) I felt like the floodgates opened and that I joined some sort of "battered babies" speakeasy. What was worse, these parents were harboring so much guilt that it was eating them alive inside!

We have to take proper safety precautions and use our heads, but we can't let ourselves get too crazy and riddled with guilt or we'll miss out on the fun along the way.

With regards to spending time with your baby, let me explain before it sounds like I'm contradicting myself from last chapter. We're redefining normal that you are NOT a monster for needing a break from your baby every so often. When you take that break, you should be doing it guilt-free. You can't be together 24 hours per day, 7 days per week, 52 weeks per year. Technically, you can, but I wouldn't recommend it. You'll get batty, and your baby will never get to know the other loving, caring humans in his or her life.

This was by far the biggest source of my mom guilt, which is absolutely ridiculous when you stop to think about it. I worked from home, my baby slept with me, and I had done the best I could to adjust my work time around his sleeping time. However, what I found was that I wasn't leaving any time for me. Even the most energized of Energizer bunnies needs a little time to recharge.

Mamas, you need you time. It is a totally exhausting job being a mom. I don't care if you're a stay-at-home mom, a mom with a nanny and two very involved grandmas, a working mom, or whatever. Looking after a little one during the first few years when they are completely dependent on you wears on you emotionally, mentally, and physically. And, if you've been a rebel like me and you're breastfeeding, bedsharing, etc., there is little time apart.

I'm giving you an invitation to TAKE TIME FOR YOURSELF as often as you need to. That may be once per day at first, and THAT IS OKAY. That doesn't make you weak or a crappy mom. That means you know your limits, and when your battery is low you need to recharge. If you want to sit on the couch when your baby naps and binge watch the latest Netflix craze because you know you'll feel more alive when your baby wakes up, DO IT. The laundry and the dust will always be there.

For others, taking time for yourself may be once per week or once per month. Whatever it is, take the time. Find someone else to look after your baby. Even if you're a single mom, when there's a will there's a way. I don't know who said those words of wisdom, but it's another classic quote to live by. You will not believe how much better you feel when you take the time you need. The better you feel, the better mama you are. The better mama you are, the happier, more content your baby is. The happier, more content your baby is, the more enjoyable a time you will have together. And all of a sudden, you may not need to recharge your battery as often as you used to. Do you see how this works?

Okay, time to school those three monkeys. In my humble opinion, when it comes to what babies hear, it's not so much what you say but how you say it. If I haven't made this point by now, babies are incredibly intuitive little beings. They pick up on tone of voice and inflections. If you're always stressed, speaking in that super annoying high-pitched "clean your mess up" mom tone, baby is going to feel that anxiety and stress. Similarly, if you're always speaking with humor and joy, you're probably still using a super annoying high-pitched mom tone, but it's the "you're so cute, I love you so much" tone, the one that makes baby feel happy and safe. Does this sound like common sense? Good, because it is. Use your head; keep the fights, stress, and anxiety conversations for when baby is not around and fast asleep. You're the adult in this situation, so act like one. Better yet, ditch those conversations altogether. Ain't no one got time to be miserable when there is a baby to tend to!

When baby sees evil: Another really fun piece of parenting advice to try to navigate through is when and how much is appropriate screen time. There are many guidelines out there, and yeah, you guessed it, plenty of conflicting points of view. I'm going to be a big rebel for a minute and recommend that instead of sifting through it all, how about we just stop the screen time? Like seriously, enough with the phones, computers, and TVs in front of baby when we can help it. We all could benefit from a little digital detox, am I right?

I'll share with you this little nugget from the AAP: "Children younger than 2 years need hands-on exploration and social interaction with trusted caregivers to develop their cognitive, language, motor, and social-emotional skills. Because of their immature symbolic, memory, and attentional skills, infants and toddlers cannot learn from traditional digital media as they do from interactions with caregivers, and they have difficulty transferring that knowledge to their 3-dimensional experience. The chief factor that facilitates toddlers' learning from commercial media (starting around 15 months of age) is parents watching with them and reteaching the content."[1] You know what I just read there? Don't regularly plop your toddler in front of a TV or hand them a tablet or iPhone and walk away. Doing it every once in a while, however, to allow yourself the opportunity to empty the dishwasher (which is actually a fun task to include your mobile tot in) or make it through the grocery store checkout line without a meltdown, should not result in mom guilt.

I'm going to call myself out on the floor for a minute. I used to judge parents when I'd be out to eat and see their little ones glued to tablets or smartphones. I'd think things like "so neglectful" or "get a babysitter". What a pretentious naïve snob I was! These poor parents were just trying to feel like real people, having someone else cook and clean up for them for one night and attempt some adult conversation! For all I knew, all other nights they ate together as a family and talked to each other without any screens in sight. Looking back, I should have applauded those rebels, completely boycotting the mom (and dad) guilt!

Speaking of eating, the third evil—taste no evil—is constantly giving mamas the guilt. We already talked about food in chapter six, but it bears repeating in the context of rebelling against the mom guilt.

Do not obsess about the "bad" foods your baby is exposed to on occasion or go out of your way to make foods forbidden. Try to play it cool even if you're horrified by what your baby is consuming. Don't make it into a big deal, and it won't be a big deal. Babies and toddlers are super tuned into your responses and will pick up on the most subtle cues (or the not-so-subtle cue of you scrunching up your face in disgust). Sure, your cousin just gave your 13-month-old half of her ice cream cone right before nap time and you're now bracing yourself for the sugar rush that is going to screw up all things sleep, but once in a while isn't going to turn into ice cream for three meals per day. I promise. And, you're not a terrible mother for allowing your tot to indulge in an apple cider doughnut with daddy on a crisp fall day. In fact, one would argue you're a little bit of a killjoy if you don't.

The reality is that a cookie is just a cookie. While it might taste good, it's not going to WOW baby, unless you make a big deal about the cookie being so good and so amazing. Then the cookie becomes more than a cookie: it becomes an experience, something that makes mommy (or more likely, grandma) happy. Baby LOVES to make others happy, and so the tradition of junk food for pleasure continues and is passed down to baby's generation. Don't feel guilty about the occasional treat, just be prepared for the potential explosive poop or rock-hard constipated belly that could be on the other end of that splurge. Even small dietary changes of Jack's have always greeted me with a "throw out these pants they're ruined" poop or a "am I going to have to stick my hand up there and yank out that rock" bout of constipation.

WHAT WORKED FOR ME

It took me a while to come to terms with the fact that the driveway fall was just an accident, and accidents happen. Even to this day, I catch myself starting to go down that dark hole of what ifs, and I have to pull myself out, reminding myself that I have to let it go. I don't know if I would have ever been able to forgive myself if something permanent resulted from it, but I finally came to the realization that lamenting over it wasn't doing me any good.

I can't wrap him in bubble wrap, as much I'd like to, and I learned that even when holding him, accidents could happen. I've tried to lighten up since then, and some days are easier than others. There were still certain activities that Jack did that I dubbed "Do those with Daddy", like climbing the slide ladder at the park. Justin is incredibly careful with Jack, and I feel comfortable if I leave the two of them alone while they run around outside or climb things that make my pulse quicken and sweat to bead on my forehead even in the dead of winter.

As much as I enjoy my time with Jack, I'm going to share a secret with you: I've watched the clock and counted down until nap time or until Daddy comes home or whatever time was going to give me a few minutes of peace. And, I've felt bad about it, just like I'm sure you do too. In today's day and age when all you see are pictures and video clips of happy moms with smiling babies, you're often left to wonder if you're the only one who just needs five flipping seconds to themselves. You're not. I just told you I'm obsessed with my child, and I've still done the "watch the clock" thing. It is OKAY. There is nothing to feel guilty over for needing a break. Anyone who tells you they've never done it, watch their nose grow as they tell you that lie.

I remember during the pandemic that I had a coworker who came over for a happy hour on a Friday night during the summer. She stayed for about ninety minutes, sixty of which was just us on the back deck and the other thirty we played with Jack. We chatted about work, personal lives, food, etc. We drank a little bit of wine, and we enjoyed a few snacks. After she left, I felt elated. I immediately said to my husband, "You should try to get a golf game on the calendar with your friends before it gets too cold out." We don't always realize we need it, but the time to unwind and recharge is invaluable.

As cute as those three little monkeys are, their advice is not practical when it comes to shielding our babies from all things evil. The mom guilt we bestow upon ourselves as a result is also impractical.

I've made a conscious effort to clean up my vocabulary, but I'm also not going to stress over it. There should be no mom guilt if my baby's first word is shit (which it wasn't). It's not my fault, though, that it's an incredibly easy word for a baby learning to talk to say. If people didn't want babies to pick up on cusses, then supercalifragilisticexpialidocious should have been used instead of "shit".

Here's my rule of thumb with the treats at our house: Food is more of an exploratory opportunity to touch, smell, see, and taste. Babies aren't all that interested in food for purposes of consumption unless they're really hungry. Babies haven't developed the super frustrating and unattractive habits that we adults have, where we mindlessly eat or eat to numb whatever is tweaking us that day. What gets them excited and cures them from whatever is tweaking them is YOU, not a chocolate chip cookie.

This is a hard concept for parents to grasp because almost all of us are excited by a chocolate chip cookie (like, I want one right now after simply typing that sentence) and that's because of our prior experiences with said chocolate chip cookie and the habits we've formed.

Rebelling against mom guilt was probably the hardest thing for me to do, harder than deciding to let Jack into my bed or nurse him well past a year. I still struggle with this one and have to consciously put in effort to be badass here. Remember my thoughts earlier about taking care of all of you? The "all" part includes our mental sanity! We have to let the mom guilt go! Our baby loves us in the purest way, the way all love strives to be but oftentimes falls short.

I've made Jack a priority, and I will continue to make him a priority. Pandemic or not, I didn't have as many social events planned, and the ones I did have usually involved him being there too. It's imperative, though, that you make the time to keep you, you.

How do you know if you're nailing it? It's not a mystery, Mama. Your baby will tell you. They're not one to hold in their feelings, as you might have noticed. If they're discontent or hurt or scared, you'll know you've got to make an adjustment somewhere. If they're generally well, then stop the nail-biting fear that you're screwing it all up. Be full of care but free of worry. These first few years are short; don't stress them away. You'll miss the magical moments in between.

Right now, I am a better mom than I am a wife. I am a better mom than I am employee. I am a better mom than I am daughter, sister, and friend. Balance in life is not about holding all roles equally at all times; it's about knowing when to step up which roles. So, be a better mom than any other role in these early days and do so unapologetically.

I've released the ability to feel that I'm being a terrible mom and recognized I cannot control it all. This pains me to admit, no matter how many times I've admitted it by now. There will be accidents, mommy timeouts, swear words, screen time, and ice cream sundaes that I'm not a failure because of. I've decided I'm a better mom because of them. They remind me that I'm human, not a machine. Being human is a beautiful thing. It means I'm alive and allowing myself to truly be.

9

Imperfect is the New Perfect
Perfection

ROAD TO REBELLION

I was not immune to the social media scroll. Do you realize how frequently new moms are breastfeeding? Since you know I'm not a TV girl, I was limited to activities I could do on my phone when I wanted to pass the time. I found myself obsessing over other moms' posts who had babies around the same time Jack was born. There were two in particular I remember, and I was subconsciously constantly comparing. I'd find myself quietly gloating when Jack reached a milestone, like crawling, earlier. Then, I'd find myself biting my bottom lip when I'd see "She slept 8 hours straight last night, and mama feels great!" posts, worried that there might be something wrong with Jack for still waking up all damn night.

There was judging, there was pity, there was envy, there was victory, and there was so much wasted time and wasted mental energy. These people are LOOSE acquaintances, not my best friends or family, and yet I knew the daily happenings of their lives, or at least I felt like I did. Then there are the people who REALLY put it out there. We're taking deep dark postpartum depression feelings, sleep deprivation announcements, and cries for help. It's intense and can make you uncomfortable for knowing so much about someone you know nothing else about.

While the in-person gatherings may have halted, I still had access to the entire world of mamas and babies, bombarding me with their day's trials and tribulations, all at the tap of a button. Before I knew it, I had this false sense of what a perfect baby or a perfect mama was supposed to look like.

This need to have a perfect image starts on day one. Pre-baby, even pre-pregnancy, I never understood the professional photograph sessions families would have in the hospital. Since when did your stay at the hospital turn into an amusement park ride...where your photo is taken at some random point on the ride and then strategically displayed to you in a cute souvenir frame on your way out the door, just begging you to buy it? Post-baby, I was FLOORED that women could pull themselves together for these photos.

You heard my story, I was fortunate for a relatively short, easy delivery with a fast recovery. If anyone should have been able to pull it together for a photo shoot, it should have been me. But, is that real life? Full transparency: I went into the hospital with day-old hair, and I left the hospital never having washed it. I was wearing disposable underwear (who knew such a thing existed) and a maxi pad that could have doubled as a mattress for a small dog. A photo shoot wasn't exactly on the top of my priority list.

That's just the beginning. How about the parent and baby matching outfits or the adorable newborn shots of the baby in a laundry basket or flower bed? It's easy to assume that these people have it all together, and there must be something wrong with you because your hair is piled up on the top of your head and looks as though it could double as a bird's nest, and you're not sure if your T-shirt is dirty or clean, never mind if it matches your baby's attire. Jack was born in the middle of summer. We basically lived topless, him in a diaper and me in a nursing top with my girls hanging out. I have endless pictures of THAT if you're interested.

Then, there are the monthly birthday photos—which you're obligated to take, of course, because you received at your baby shower several plaques, blocks, blankets, stickers, bows, and bowties to use as props for these pictures. I did this every month for the first year, and I think Jack cooperated for exactly one photo of one month. The rest are either blurry, his eyes are closed, or he's half in the picture.

Before I even had Jack, I had been to many first birthday parties, all of which had me scratching my head in confusion and mentally tallying up the pretty pennies spent on such elaborate affairs. A petting zoo, one hundred of your closest friends, a cake that looks like it should be in a Saks Fifth Avenue window display, SO MANY gifts, piñatas, ice cream trucks, clowns, and the list goes on and on. Meanwhile, the guest of honor spends ninety percent of the event sleeping, crying, or eating, and ten percent of the event interested in how the cake smashes and how the wrapping paper crinkles. In addition, mommy and daddy (or sometimes grandma and grandpa) are out thousands of dollars and are absolutely exhausted.

It wasn't just about comparing Jack to other babies. There was also subtle marriage comparison too. I can remember my jaw dropping at parents of babies constantly on date nights out and weekend getaways. Trust me, Justin and I love a good night out, we certainly had many of them before becoming parents. Tripping the light fantastic was something we knew and loved but also something we figured would be limited once we became parents. We just didn't realize quite how limited.

My parents were gracious enough to offer to watch Jack again after our first successful night out, around when he was four and a half months old. This time didn't go as well. We came back, and my dad had so much baby snot on his shirt, a telltale sign that Jack cried the ENTIRE time.

On Valentine's Day, Jack at seven months of age, we wised up a bit. We decided we'd do the early bird special and have dinner early so that we'd be home before bed, just a short two-hour dinner close by home. My sister was in town, and we were gone for an hour before the text messages started coming in. They started out with "he seems fussy" and quickly escalated to "please wrap up your food and get home ASAP". We walked into the house, hearing Jack whimpering, and found my sister, Marissa, standing in front of the fridge, double doors wide open, Jack propped in her arms. Perhaps hoping Mommy was hidden behind the ketchup bottle? (What is it with the cold air and people thinking that'll calm this boy down?!)

These "relaxing" date nights required dressing in real clothes (or just dressing, period). This was always when I'd hold my breath and hope my breastfeeding snacking hadn't impacted my ability to button my jeans. Postpartum body image issues are real, my dear.

I was probably about six months postpartum when one day my husband slapped my ass and said, "Whoa, we better put that in the freezer to firm up." Now, you might read that and automatically get defensive on my part, and I love you for that, but surprisingly I wasn't insulted or mad. I actually laughed hysterically. He was so right. Even though I was back down to my pre-baby weight and wearing my pre-baby clothes (proudly) and I was working out regularly (squats and all), my butt was still SO SOFT. I even took Jack for at least a forty-five minute walk every day. It was naptime for him and fresh air time for me! I told myself the jiggle was because my body was using my derrière as fat storage for Jack's breastmilk, and I rocked that Jell-O butt with pride.

My husband and I are fiercely competitive. I'm not kidding, we've had nights where we played an innocent card game, I win, he'll sulk the rest of the evening, and then the next morning tell me why I got "lucky" and what hands he didn't get lucky on that cost him the game. From an outsider view, I have to imagine it's both comical and intimidating to witness. (It speaks volumes that even in the example I give about how we're competitive, it's a time when I won). So, naturally any time we were exposed to other families and their small tots, he was comparing and sizing them up against Jack.

Jack wasn't much interested in other people for the first eight months of his life, and then after that he was stuck at home quarantining. As a total introvert myself, I secretly find it one of his most enduring traits. We'd see other babies and toddlers easily interacting with others, happy to be held by a total stranger, and Justin would say to me afterwards how we have to get him more socialized and around more people. (This is pre-pandemic, mind you, so we cannot even blame social distancing and quarantining for Jack's disinterest in making friends.) Even so, I internally started gnawing on the idea that maybe he does need to get out more, yet externally I stood my ground and proclaimed that there is nothing wrong with him. Every person is different, and we don't have to adjust who he's exposed to just because he's not reacting to other people as openly as the children we were socializing with.

Because of Jack's low birth weight, I tended to obsess over his weight for the first few months of his life. I'd weigh myself, then go get Jack and weigh myself again with him in my arms, subtract the difference (and silently thank the heavens that I didn't weigh that much anymore) and immediately plug it into an online baby percentile calculator to make sure he was still tracking in the 40th-50th percentile (which he always was).

A good friend of mine was distraught that her eighteen-month-old daughter didn't have enough words in her vocabulary, according to her pediatrician. Apparently, she should be saying at least twenty-five words, and she barely had ten that were coming out coherently. My girlfriend was as obsessive about her daughter's words as I was about Jack's weight. She kept a list in the kitchen to track her words. She was fearful she'd be forced to take her to a speech therapist. Forced, as if that was actually something she couldn't say, "Buzz off. I'll decide that."

REDEFINING NORMAL

We are mothering in some bizarre times, and I'm not just saying that because I wrote this book during a pandemic. Social media has made life gnarly. What may have started out with good intentions, hoping to connect those around the world to one another, has now become the ultimate comparison and competition platform.

People thought keeping up with the Joneses was difficult in the 20th century. That was nothing compared to today, leveraging social media and being able to connect with and see an infinite number of people, how they want us to perceive how they live their lives, and then us ultimately trying to live up to those standards. I'm pretty sure our nervous systems weren't meant for all this scrolling. It's here and it's real and it 100% impacts how we mother.

Deranged and distorted come to mind as two words to describe the perception that is created by social media. We like to use terms like "hot mess" to indicate our shit isn't together, while really trying to show off some version of ourselves that is very much flattering. I saw a post once of a woman who was showing us her true self, "unfiltered", and she looked like she was modeling for a lingerie catalog. (Are catalogs even still a thing?) Social media is riddled with contrary concepts that lead us to think so-and-so lives this perfect life and has wonderful children who are always happy and a loving husband who is always there for them.

Have I mentioned yet that new moms are really vulnerable? It's not uncommon during the first few weeks of your baby's life to feel like the best mom on the planet, the biggest failure to ever see the light of day, the world's fattest cow, and the most beautiful lady in all the land all within a two-hour span. All it takes is a few postpartum hormones and a scroll through your newsfeed to set that emotional roller coaster in motion.

What we forget is that we see the version of others' lives they want us to see, and it is information overload. It can negatively impact the way we mother whether we want to admit it or not. I had to force myself to stop. If you need someone to force you, too, here you go: Stop comparing. Just stop.

You start to feel like an obsessive stalker. Motivational speaker Jim Rohn is known for proclaiming, "You're the average of the top five people you spend the most time with." While we're not literally spending time with these people on social media, we're more influenced by them than we realize. Who are the top five people you're watching? Are they positive influences? Our self-esteem, way of thinking, and decision making are all impacted by those we are exposed to every day.

I recognize it's not all bad. Sure, you know way more about the twin girls the mousy blonde from high school home room raised than you do your own sister, but if you leverage social media to follow inspirational influencers or to stay in touch with friends and family around the world, it can be a positive experience. However, it should not consume us, and we should limit the time we spend scrolling.

I am all about the pictures. There is nothing cuter in this world than a baby. (I'm not a pet person at all, so unfortunately your dogs and cats do nothing for me). Let's take photos and take lots of them. If there is one thing we have as new moms that's easier than any generation of new moms before us, it's the ability to snap a pic. It's effortless. You don't have to develop the film, date the photo, and spend three minutes per picture trying to separate the plastic slot in a photo album to catalog them. You'll want them later on in life, and so will your children. But, they don't all have to be worthy of entry into the Gerber Baby contest. In fact, the candid ones are nine times out of ten better than the staged ones. And, you don't have to share them with anyone if you don't want to or have to post them on any app—especially the ones you're in, where your hair looks like you just poured a bottle of Italian dressing over your head.

Which brings me to my next point of rebellion: your appearance. It is OKAY that we have days (possibly in a row) where we don't shower. If we do shower, we probably will rarely style our hair. There is nothing glamorous or red carpet-like about motherhood. You will be covered in spit up, mustard colored poop, and breast milk for months.

It's also not guaranteed that your body is going to bounce back. In fact, your body may never be the same, and that is beautiful. Even if you are one of those lucky bitches who are back in their pre-baby jeans two weeks after the hospital, there are scars, stretch marks, swollen boobs, wider hips, new face creases, and more grey hairs. These are all badges on honor that you should look at with pride, not with disgust. Mama, you grew a human being and brought that little ball of life into this world. It is so mind-blowingly amazing, and the physical changes that come along with it are too.

Give yourself grace. Do not calorie deplete (especially if you're breastfeeding). You need all the energy you can get. Treat your insides with kindness and fuel your body with nutritious foods, and eventually you'll find your ideal weight. Also, treat your soul with kindness and eat a chocolate bar every so often...but not every day. If you do eat one every day, acknowledge it. Let's not lament over not being the same size we were before baby if we're drowning our postpartum sorrows in a pint of ice cream every night, okay?

And, for the love of all things good, move. Move that body. It doesn't have to be a sixty-minute cardio class every day (ain't no one got time for that). Our bodies weren't meant to act like slugs. Movement helps our insides (circulation, digestion, muscles) and our outsides (love handles, muffin tops, flappy arms—or in my case, Jell-O butt).

Not hating your spouse can get challenging in that first year of motherhood, even if you do laugh along when they call attention to your booty imperfections. It's easy to forget life back when you were making "table for two" reservations. I have a secret though; going out to dinner isn't the only way to carve out time for your marriage. We don't have to plan nights on the town with our husbands. And, we certainly don't have to do that if it's to the detriment of our mental health. I tip my hat to you, Mama, if you're able to leave your baby for long periods of time and there are no meltdowns. It's impressive to me, but if it doesn't work for your circumstances, why force it? It's not good for you, for baby, and most definitely not for grandma and grandpa (and auntie). Instead, let's change the way we view date night.

Date night can be a relaxing bath together, a massage, or a home-cooked meal that you eat late at night when baby is asleep. Hell, date night can be snuggling up and binge watching an entire season of Schitt's Creek (because you are extra-terrestrial if you can stop at one episode). Find time to be husband and wife (and not mommy and daddy), but do it in a way that doesn't cause you stress. If you're stressed and distracted, that defeats the purpose of spending time together to focus on you as a couple.

The first birthday parties. Where to even start? The last time I checked, people have no conscious memories of age one. And, babies certainly don't have the strength nor hand-eye coordination to swing at a piñata. Also, if you were paying attention at all during chapter six, they have no need for frosted cake. Mama, if the idea of throwing a first birthday party has your stomach in knots and your arm pits sweating, REBEL. Sign off Pinterest, cancel your Party City shopping cart, and call off the ponies. Tell your mother-in-law tough shit if her college best friend wanted to meet your baby. (The same friend she demanded was invited to your wedding and who spent the entire time taking advantage of the open bar and flirting with the DJ, hoping he would take advantage of her.) The only thing you need to do on that special day is congratulate yourself and honor the experience you had one year ago, bringing your baby into the world.

Before you get your panties all in a bunch, if you are jazzed by professional newborn photos or first birthday parties, by all means, do it up, Mama! The beautiful thing about motherhood is it's YOUR journey, so forge your path ahead. A dear friend of mine had twins, and after I had Jack, she shared with me that every single day of her maternity leave she woke up, showered, and put on makeup. It wasn't for selfies or for her husband or her baby boys. It was for HER. It made her feel normal, like she had something in this scary and overwhelming world under control, even if it was just her eyeliner pen. We need to remember to support each other. As mamas, do what makes you feel good inside. If you only focus on doing what makes you look good on the outside, you're going to find this motherhood journey to be the biggest uphill battle of your life. Please, dear friend, rebel with me against the comparison and the jealousy and the gloating. None of that is a good look anyway.

Can we talk about milestones for a hot second? Let's start with the good. Generally speaking, it comes with good intent when you attend your baby's doctor appointments and they ask questions about rolling, standing, walking, talking, etc. The same goes for weight, height, and head size. There are certain signs they're looking for to determine if your baby is or isn't progressing appropriately. It's not to make you feel bad if you have a late bloomer, nor is it to give you bragging rights for how advanced your baby Einstein is. It's simply a precautionary way to identify any early indications of a possible issue.

These are also not milestones to hang your hat on. Think about it. Has anyone recently asked you whether you started walking at eleven months or fourteen months? And, if you answered, "fourteen months," did they judge you? Of course not! What about whether you said ten words or twenty-five words at eighteen months? Would they laugh in your face if you answer, "ten words"? Sounds absurd, doesn't it? Your destiny is not determined by whether you're a prodigy or a late bloomer as a tot.

For the record, I didn't walk until I was fourteen months old because my mom was neurotic and carried me everywhere out of fear I'd fall and hurt myself. Miraculously, this fact did not limit the number of college acceptances I got senior year of high school. So, if it doesn't matter when you're old and grown, why is there such a spotlight on it in the moment?

Does anyone ever stop to think that perhaps all of these preconceived notions of how we're programmed to think we're supposed to be might be impacting how so many mamas struggle to adjust to motherhood? Of course, sleep deprivation and hormone changes are largely to blame, but if we went into this journey without any prior knowledge, only our natural-born instincts to guide the way, do you think photo shoots and piñatas would be where we'd land? I'd venture to guess we might be more at peace, living in the moment, taking cues from our baby instead of from our news feed on how to proceed each day.

WHAT WORKED FOR ME

I ended up replacing much of the time I spent on social media apps with my Kindle (because I have yet to master being able to hold either a sleeping or a nursing baby while reading a physical book with two hands. I'm just not that talented and never will be). I used the time to fulfill one of my favorite pastimes, reading...which then shifted into fulfilling one of my other favorite pastimes, writing. Now, here we are.

I also had to break up with Google. Typing anything that resembles "8-month-old won't [fill in the blank] - normal?" is a recipe for disaster. You will find just as many hits to answer "yes" as you will to answer "no", and you'll go insane.

If you're feeling overwhelmed and have an unhealthy relationship with your smartphone, put it down. It doesn't make you weird or an addict that you don't feel good about how you're using social media. It doesn't make you weak that the pressures of creating this perfect life story feel impossible. I'm right there with you, and there are more of us out there than you'd think. You're not alone in these thoughts that being perfect is completely unachievable.

Not only is a perfect image unachievable, but it's also unrealistic. Life happens. Murphy's Law exists for a reason. Plans get screwed up. Motherhood is no exception. Own it. Yet it is the one area that women try the HARDEST to be perfect.

My blow dryer went untouched for months when Jack was first born, and I think I applied mascara twice in the first three months. When COVID-19 hit, I essentially had no reason to pull myself together or leave the house for a long time (which was such a relief to not have to subject Jack or my family to anymore disastrous date nights).

I love Justin more in parenthood than I did before we were parents. In retrospect, date nights weren't what fostered that love. Surviving parenthood together, carving out time for each other at random times each day, laughing with him or at him until I peed my pants (because, oh yeah, that's now a thing) is what made my marriage stronger and more fruitful. We never did an overnight away, just the two of us, and miraculously we stayed married! I kid, but I am saying that the perfect marriage is just as insane of a concept as the perfect mother. I've wanted to draw on his face with a Sharpie when he was peacefully sleeping at 2 a.m. and I was nursing Jack for the fifth time that night, and I know for a fact he's wanted to lock me up in the toy chest when he's tripped over a plastic train Jack and I left in the middle of the floor.

I was fortunate enough that Jack's first birthday fell during the pandemic, so his "party" was an intimate gathering of seven, including him. I would have done it the same way without COVID-19, though. I'm sure I would have pissed off a few people, but by now they're used to me. I basked in the warm sun. I recounted that beautiful day 366 days ago and all the ups and downs, laughing, and crying. I ate about one-third of Jack's cake during his afternoon nap. (He had zero interest in his birthday cake and all the interest in the world in his balloons). It was a fantastic day, celebrating with the people I love the most, and it cost me less than $100.

Somewhere around six or seven months of age, I stopped weighing Jack regularly. I finally had to have a "come to Jesus" with myself and stop the madness. It's hard, though. As a mama, anything that isn't tracking as "normal" you instantly blame yourself for. I get it, and I've been there.

What I came to realize was that in your baby's eyes, you are perfect. That is truly all that matters during those early days. You're not a great mom because your two-inch-by-two-inch digital squares are picture perfect. You're a great mom for putting your baby first (and by first, I mean before a hot shower or a warm meal).

Your house will be dirty, your laundry will pile up, and you will run out of food to eat. This is real motherhood. We've got to get the Hollywood and Instagram images out of our heads. Instead, rebel against the image of perfect, and embrace how perfect your imperfect world truly is.

"Authenticity is the daily practice of letting go of who we think we're supposed to be and embracing who we are," Brené Brown with the mic drop.

Conclusion

No matter which path you forge, it's inevitable that you'll find yourself doubting your decisions at times, even if you followed your gut 100% of the time. I have many accounts of when I wondered if I made the right call, even though felt in my heart I did. We're all human, susceptible to insecurities and doubt! No one is perfect (refer back to chapter 9), and I'm so far from it that it's comical. Not that I regret any of my decisions, but I've absolutely doubted myself from time to time. (I'm a firm believer in having no regrets in life, just lessons learned.) Parenting is a constant stream of paranoia woven with a constant stream of heart-swelling love, beautifully twisted.

When Jack was about five months old, I changed his diaper one day after work and saw something white at the tip of his penis. I wiped and it came right off, so I didn't think much about it, in a rush to get him changed and get dinner on the table.

The next night, roughly around the same time, Justin was on diaper duty, and shouted from the changing table, "Laura come here!" I went running in, worried something is wrong. He said, "Look at this." Sure enough, the same whiteness I saw the day before was there. I said, "Yes, I saw something like that yesterday." Alarmed, he proclaimed, "You did?! You didn't tell me!" and I said, "Well, I was in a hurry, and it came right off."

Horrified, he looked at me and said, "This is serious. I think he has a UTI. This is what we have to be prepared for because we didn't circumcise him. I know guys from hockey that have had this."

Feeling guilty for dismissing it so quickly the previous day, I texted my dad to ask if he noticed anything like what Justin and I were seeing. He said he hadn't seen anything white, but he had seen some diaper rash so he's been putting Desitin on him. I started laughing.

Justin, now seeing me laughing, got even more worked up and asked me what was so funny. (How could I possibly be laughing during a 911 crisis?)

"I think that's just some Desitin we're seeing." You know, the white cream that smeared on the top of his penis when his diaper was closed up, that wipes off easily. The nerve of Desitin masquerading around my son's manhood as a urinary tract infection!

There are moments where your ignorance and naïvety are going to shine. Sometimes they will be laughable, oftentimes you may blush when reminiscing for years to come. Jack's first official pediatrician appointment was one of those times. I was a complete and total train wreck, but two distinct moments will haunt me for a long time. The first is when I told the pediatrician that we didn't circumcise Jack (in a hushed tone, as if the walls had ears and were judging me). I quickly followed up that statement with asking, "So, how do we wash it?" as if an intact penis required special care. Bless his soul, he respectfully answered, "Like any other body part, a little soap and water."

Mortified, I simply nodded and started babbling about something else.

Shortly after asking about the penis washing, while holding Jack in my arms, I felt and heard him take a huge smash in his diaper. Panic took over my body. The doctor hadn't yet examined Jack, and I had no diapers or wipes with me. Trying to play it cool, I laughed and made some lame joke about the doctor giving Jack the nervous poops. The doctor laughed it off and told me not to worry and that I could go ahead and change him. Yes, yes, I wish I could. I admitted I had nothing with me, and he produced some wipes from the exam room cabinet and then called his nurse for a diaper. They only had a larger-sized diaper, which looked absolutely ridiculous on Jack's little six-pound frame. It's a miracle he didn't called social services on us right then and there, looking like the most unfit parents in that moment.

As human beings, we have conscious thoughts and are cognitive beings. It's what makes us the dominant species (that and our opposable thumbs) and puts us at the top of the animal kingdom. This is both a blessing and a curse, and we're cursed badly when it comes to modern parenting. Seriously, I'd give anything to be an elephant for the first year of motherhood. Elephants don't have to do months of mental preparation for childbirth; they just push that thing out. There are no lactation consultants on call in the safari. Dumbo just latches! There are snuggles at night and nursing until it doesn't feel needed and intact penises and zero expectations that mama elephant looks like a catalog model within three months of delivery. Plus, I would seriously crush peanuts morning, noon, and night if I got to be an elephant for a year.

Because my elephant fantasy is completely unrealistic and I'm stuck with this nonstop-thinking brain, I've realized that the only way to unlearn what we've been told is to think less, feel more, and then relearn what we feel is perfectly acceptable. Not only is it perfectly acceptable, but there are also so many people on this quest, lifting up the covers of history and humanity and science and evolution and finding that it's not weird or creepy or gross. It's biologically expected and programmed into us. Fight through the societal programming, and rewire your brain. Rebel against modern norms, and be the elephant you never knew you always wanted to be! Reconnect with biological norms, and disconnect from cultural norms.

Culture influences our thinking, what we normalize, and our expectations. We have to acknowledge that. This book would be dull and boring in some cultures. The title would be *Basic Mama*, and it would be the equivalent of reading a book about tasks like brushing our teeth, boiling a pot of water, and taking out the garbage because the topics covered in here are still much ingrained in some cultures.

My thoughts on the ways to mother Jack were so different before Jack was born. We need to remind ourselves that it's okay if we do a complete 180 once we're mamas, on anything as big as how long we breastfeed for or as little as which baby carrier we use. I'm still dizzy from how many times I spun from one way to another way on so many topics.

Sometimes we just need reassurance. In a world where there are so many rules that go against what we feel, it's understandable to be torn and conflicted. The only way I could find reassurance was to dig, read, and discover. I envision a world where that isn't the case, where everyone is kinder and more open and more in tune with one another. Let this book be one step towards that motherhood utopia.

Motherhood made me human. I feel more, I listen internally more, I am humble and vulnerable and scared and overjoyed and bone-tired. I've been wrong, I've been right, and I found out that oftentimes there is no wrong or right. There are more than fifty shades of grey when it comes to becoming a mama. All of it is so perfectly amazing. Putting it down on paper and finding all this factual validation behind my mommy sixth sense was so cathartic. Sharing this revelation with you turned out to be more therapeutic for my transformation from rule-follower than any psychiatrist session ever could have been.

If you make decisions that align with your gut, and not with a rule book, you're not a failure—you're a rebel. If you are called a failure, tell that sorry soul that you're happy to fail the meaningless standards that society has created for new moms.

Parenting can be challenging. Attachment parenting especially can wear down the Pollyanna-est of us all. I've completely bought into the theory, though, that attachment parenting is a short-term investment for long-term gain. All the love and nurturing and dependency will create a confident, happy human. I can't prove it to be true (yet), but it's a bet I'm willing to make. Dare I throw one last quote your way? "It is easier to build strong children than to repair broken men." —Frederick Douglass

No more lying to our doctors, no more lying to family and friends, and most importantly no more lying to ourselves. Trust yourself and do you, Mama. Tattoo the truth to your soul, spray paint your freedom as graffiti. Throw away the rule book. Be a rebel mama.

XOXO

1

Epilogue

That burning sensation every time he would nurse...I ignored it for a day, assumed I made it up in my head or that he was just latching funny. Then, on the second day it was a little harder to ignore, and I admitted to myself, "Okay, it's pretty painful when he nurses." Then, in the bathroom when I wiped myself, "Oh no, is that milky discharge on the toilet paper?"

On the third day I conclude FML; I have thrush. I couldn't deny that the pain in my nipples must be from the infection and the discharge I saw on the toilet paper from the vaginal yeast infection.

"How did this happen?" I asked out loud to no one in particular. I kicked myself for not washing my hands enough and I was annoyed at myself for not changing Jack's diaper more frequently (even though rarely did he go more than three to four hours in a given day without a diaper change). I figured as a result of my neglectful parenting, he probably developed a little yeast from a wet diaper. I must have touched it when changing him and spread it to myself.

I spent the next twenty-four hours obsessively checking his mouth for white patches and observing his behavior for fussiness when he nursed, neither of which I found. On the hottest setting of the washing machine, I washed every towel, sheet, and article of clothing either of us had recently worn. I all but wrapped the two of us in ClingWrap to avoid further spread. The irony of surviving without contracting COVID-19 through the pandemic only to be met with another fast-spreading infection, was not lost on me. Too busy cleaning the house, I put off calling the doctor for a remedy until the next day.

I never ended up needing to make that phone call. I woke up the following morning, headed to the bathroom, and found a much different treat on my toilet paper. There staring back at me, all pretty and pink, was my first postpartum period, just a few days shy of Jack's eighteen-month birthday.

I was flabbergasted. I knew that as you wean from breastfeeding your body regulates and your period returns, but I assumed since Jack still nursed around the clock I hadn't gotten to that point. (The longest break we had from nursing was eight hours, and that day was a goddamn unicorn. What was more common were five- to six-hour breaks.) Plus, I was still scarred from the PCOS ordeal pre-pregnancy, and a part of me worried that I wouldn't get a period again without some more blood, sweat, and tears.

I also didn't know that sore nipples, or discomfort in nipples when breastfeeding, was common amongst women anywhere from the time they ovulate leading up to their period. This is why I assumed I had thrush and why I unnecessarily deep-cleaned my entire house. Okay, fine, thrush or not, my house needed it.

Well, whoopsies for jumping to conclusions, but hooray to being thrush-free and a double-hooray for being prepared with period supplies on hand this go-round!

With my lady parts open for baby making business, I must leave you and find Justin. Time to seduce him into helping me make some sequel content. Until next time, rebel mamas!

Notes

Introduction

1. Jennifer G. Rosier and Tracy Cassels, "From 'Crying Expands the Lungs' to 'You're Going to Spoil That Baby': How the Cry-It-Out Method Became Authoritative Knowledge." *SAGE Journals* (August 13, 2020) DOI: 10.1177/0192513X20949891.

2. Lyndsey Hookway, *Holistic Sleep Coaching—Gentle Alternatives to Sleep Training: for Health & Childcare Professionals.* (Praeclarus Press, 2018).

3. Sarah J. Buckley, *Gentle Birth, Gentle Mothering: A Doctor's Guide to Natural Childbirth and Gentle Early Parenting Choices.* (Berkeley: Celestial Arts, 2009).

4. Hookway, *Holistic Sleep Coaching.*

5. Hookway, *Holistic Sleep Coaching.*

6. Sarah J. Buckley, *Gentle Birth, Gentle Mothering: The Wisdom and Science of Gentle Choices in Pregnancy, Birth, and Parenting.* (Berkeley: Celestial Arts, 2005).

7. Ina May Gaskin, *Ina May's Guide to Breastfeeding.* (Bantam, 2009).

8. Buckley, *The Wisdom and Science.*

9. Gaskin, *Ina May's Guide.*

10. Gaskin, *Ina May's Guide.*

11. Buckley, *The Wisdom and Science.*

Chapter 1

1. Dawn Stacey, PhD, "Withdrawal Bleeding from Birth Control." *Verywell Health* (May 19, 2021) https://www.verywellhealth.com/withdrawal-bleeding-906612.

2. "PCOS (Polycystic Ovary Syndrome) and Diabetes." *Centers for Disease Control and Prevention* (March 24, 2020) https://www.cdc.gov/diabetes/basics/pcos.html.

3. Neal D. Barnard, *Your Body in Balance: The New Science of Food, Hormones, and Health.* (Grand Central Publishing, 2020).

4. Clare Goodwin, *Getting Pregnant with PCOS: An Evidence-Based Approach to Treat the Root Causes of Polycystic Ovary Syndrome and Boost Your Fertility.* (Auckland: Point Publishing Limited, 2020).

5. Goodwin, *Getting Pregnant with PCOS.*

6. Goodwin, *Getting Pregnant with PCOS.*

7. Barnard, *Your Body in Balance.*

Chapter 2

1. Brendon Marotta, "American Circumcision." *IMDb.* IMDbTV. (November 11, 2017). https://www.imdb.com/title/tt7628146/.

2. David Gollaher, *Circumcision: A History of the World's Most Controversial Surgery.* (New York: Basic Books, 2021).

3. Gollaher, *Circumcision: A History.*

4. Gollaher, *Circumcision: A History.*

5. Jennifer Margulis, *The Business of Baby: What Doctors Don't Tell You, What Corporations Try to Sell You, and How to Put Your Pregnancy, Childbirth, and Baby Before Their Bottom Line.* (New York: Scribner, 2013).

6. Margulis, *The Business of Baby.*

7. Margulis, *The Business of Baby*.

8. Maria Owings, PhD, Sayeedha Uddin, MD, and Sonja Williams, MPH, "Trends in Circumcision for Male Newborns in U.S. Hospitals: 1979–2010." *Centers for Disease Control and Prevention*. (November 6, 2015) https://www.cdc.gov/nchs/data/hestat/circumcision_2013/

9. circumcision_2013.htm.

10. Susan Blank, MD and Task Force on Circumcision, "Circumcision Policy Statement." *American Academy of Pediatrics*. (September 1, 2012) DOI: 10.1542/peds.2012-1989.

11. Blank, "Circumcision Policy".

12. Carole M. Lannon and Task Force on Circumcision, "Circumcision Policy Statement." *American Academy of Pediatrics* (March 1, 1999). DOI: 10.1542/peds.103.3.686.

13. Margulis, *The Business of Baby*.

14. S. Todd Sorokan, Jane C. Finlay, and Ann L. Jefferies. "Newborn Male Circumcision: Position Statement." *Canadian Paediatric Society*. (February 2, 2021). https://www.cps.ca/en/documents/position/circumcision.

15. Billy Ray Boyd, *Circumcision Exposed: Rethinking a Medical and Cultural Tradition*. (Freedom: Crossing Press, 1998).

16. Ina May Gaskin, *Ina May's Guide to Breastfeeding*. (Bantam, 2009).

17. Margulis, *The Business of Baby*.

18. Gaskin, *Ina May's Guide*.

19. Margulis, *The Business of Baby*.

20. Margulis, *The Business of Baby*.

21. Boyd, *Circumcision Exposed*.

22. Boyd, *Circumcision Exposed*.

23. Margulis, *The Business of Baby*.

Chapter 3

1. Marie F. Mongan, *Hypnobirthing, The Mongan Method: A Natural Approach to a Safe, Easier, More Comfortable Birthing*. 4th ed. (Deerfield Beach: Health Communications, 2015).

2. Mongan, *Hypnobirthing*.

3. Barbara Harper, *Gentle Birth Choices*. (Rochester: Healing Arts Press, 2005).

4. Harper, *Gentle Birth Choices*.

5. Samantha M. Shapiro, "Mommy Wars: The Prequel." *The New York Times Magazine*. (May 23, 2012). https://www.nytimes.com/2012/05/27/magazine/ina-may-gaskin-and-the-battle-for-at-home-births.html.

6. Ina May Gaskin, *Ina May's Guide to Childbirth*. (New York: Bantam Books, 2019).

7. Diane Wiessinger, *Sweet Sleep: Nighttime and Naptime Strategies for the Breastfeeding Family*. (New York: Ballantine Books, 2014).

8. Joyce A. Martin, et al. "Births: Final Data for 2019." *National Vital Statistics Reports*. 70, no. 2. Centers for Disease Control and Prevention. (March 23, 2021). https://www.cdc.gov/nchs/data/nvsr/nvsr70/nvsr70-02-508.pdf.

9. Fay Menacker and Brady E. Hamilton. 2010. "Recent Trends in Cesarean Delivery in the United States." *NCHS Data Brief*. No. 35. Centers for Disease Control and Prevention. (March2010). https://www.cdc.gov/nchs/data/databriefs/db35.pdf.

10. Emma L. Barber, et al. "Indications Contributing to the Increasing Cesarean Delivery Rate." *U.S. National Library of Medicine* (July 2011).

11. DOI: 10.1097/AOG.0b013e31821e5f65.

12. "WHO Statement on Caesarean Section Rates." *World Health Organization*. Department of Reproductive Health and Research. (2015). http://apps.who.int/iris/bitstream/handle/10665/161442/WHO_RHR_15.02_eng.pdf;jsessionid=916A516204C52ED2104CB17458D0A6B6?sequence=1.

13. Ana Pilar Betrán, et al. "Interventions to Reduce Unnecessary Caesarean Sections in Healthy Women and Babies." *The Lancet*. (October 13, 2018). DOI: 1016/S0140-6736(18)31927-5.

14. Eva Rydahl, et al. "Cesarean Section on a Rise-Does Advanced Maternal Age Explain the Increase? A Population Register-Based Study." *National Center for Biotechnology Information Search Database*. Public Library of Science. (January 24, 2019).

15. DOI: 10.1371/journal.pone.0210655.

16. Jennifer Margulis, *The Business of Baby: What Doctors Don't Tell You, What Corporations Try to Sell You, and How to Put Your Pregnancy, Childbirth, and Baby Before Their Bottom Line*. (New York: Scribner, 2013).

17. Margulis, *The Business of Baby*.

18. Billy Ray Boyd, *Circumcision Exposed: Rethinking a Medical and Cultural Tradition*. (Freedom: Crossing Press, 1998).

19. Rebecca Dekker, "Evidence Confirms Birth Centers Provide Top-Notch Care." *American Association of Birth Centers*. (January 31, 2013). https://www.birthcenters.org/page/NBCSII.

Chapter 4

1. Tracy Gillett, *Good Science Guides: The Sleep Series*. (Raised Good, 2009).

2. Gillett, *Good Science Guides*.

3. Diane Wiessinger, *Sweet Sleep: Nighttime and Naptime Strategies for the Breastfeeding Family.* (New York: Ballantine Books, 2014).

4. Katharine Gammon, "What to Do If Your Sleep-Trained Baby Stops Sleeping." *The New York Times.* (April 17, 2020). https://www.nytimes.com/article/sleep-training-regression.html.

5. Gilda A. Morelli, et al. "Cultural Variation in Infants' Sleeping Arrangements: Questions of Independence." *Developmental Psychology* 28, no 4 (American Psychological Association, 1992). http://local.psy.miami.edu/faculty/dmessinger/c_c/rsrcs/rdgs/emot/morelli%20cosleep.dp92.pdf.

6. James J. McKenna, "Night Waking among Breastfeeding Mothers and Infants: Conflict, Congruence or Both?" *Evolution, Medicine, and Public Health*, (February 27, 2014): 40–47.

7. DOI: 10.1093/emph/eou006.

8. Ina May Gaskin, *Ina May's Guide to Breastfeeding.* (Bantam, 2009).

9. James J. McKenna, *Safe Infant Sleep: Expert Answers to Your Cosleeping Questions.* (Washington, D.C.: Platypus Media, 2020).

10. William Sears, *Nighttime Parenting: How to Get Your Baby and Child to Sleep.* (Schaumburg: La Leche League International, 1999).

11. Claire Niala, "Why African Babies Don't Cry: An African Perspective." *The Natural Child Project.* (Accessed June 25, 2021). https://www.naturalchild.org/articles/guest/claire_niala.html.

12. Sears, *Nighttime Parenting.*

13. Elizabeth Pantley, *The No-Cry Sleep Solution: Gentle Ways to Help Your Baby Sleep through the Night.* (Chicago: Contemporary Books, 2002).

14. Harvey Karp, *The Happiest Baby on the Block: The New Way to Calm Crying and Help Your Newborn Baby Sleep Longer.* 2nd ed. (New York: Bantam Books, 2015).

15. Wiessinger, *Sweet Sleep.*

Chapter 5

1. Arthur I. Eidelman and Richard J. Schanler. "Breastfeeding and the Use of Human Milk." *American Academy of Pediatrics.* (March 2012). DOI: 10.1542/peds.2011-3552.

2. "Breastfeeding." *World Health Organization.* (Accessed June 26, 2021). https://www.who.int/health-topics/breastfeeding#tab=tab_2.

3. "Cluster Feeding and Growth Spurts." *WIC Breastfeeding Support.* U.S. Department of Agriculture. (Accessed June 26, 2021). https://wicbreastfeeding.fns.usda.gov/cluster-feeding-and-growth-spurts.

4. Maija Bruun Haastrup, Anton Pottegård, and Per Damkier. "Alcohol and Breastfeeding." *Wiley Online Library.* John Wiley & Sons, Ltd. (January 4, 2014). DOI: 10.1111/bcpt.12149.

5. Diane Wiessinger, Diana West, and Teresa Pitman. *The Womanly Art of Breastfeeding.* 8th ed. (New York: Ballantine Books, 2010).

6. Jack Newman, "More Breastfeeding Myths." *Shopify.* Sympatico.ca. Handout 12. (January 2005). https://cdn.shopify.com/s/files/1/1970/0557/files/0405-more-bf-myths.pdf?13823050296189251268.

7. Haastrup, "Alcohol and Breastfeeding".

8. "Breastfeeding and Caffeine." *La Leche League International.* (June 2021). https://www.llli.org/breastfeeding-info/caffeine/.

9. Wiessinger, *The Womanly Art.*

10. Eidelman, "Use of Human Milk".

11. "Exclusive Breastfeeding for Six Months Best for Babies Everywhere." *World Health Organization*. (January 15, 2011). https://www.who.int/news/item/15-01-2011-exclusive-breastfeeding-for-six-months-best-for-babies-everywhere.

12. Katherine Dettwyler, "A Natural Age of Weaning." Department of Anthropology, Texas A&M University. (February 10, 1997). https://www.health-e-learning.com/articles/

13. A_Natural_Age_of_Weaning.pdf.

14. AAFP Breastfeeding Advisory Committee, "Breastfeeding, Family Physicians Supporting (Position Paper)." *American Academy of Family Physicians*. (2014). https://www.aafp.org/about/policies/all/breastfeeding-position-paper.html.

15. Dettwyler, "A Natural Age".

16. Mother Child. 2008. "Breast Crawl - Initiation of Breastfeeding." *YouTube*. HealthPhone™ (June 6, 2008). https://www.youtube.com/watch?v=b30Pb4WdycE.

17. Wiessinger, *The Womanly Art*.

18. Ina May Gaskin, *Ina May's Guide to Breastfeeding*. (Bantam, 2009).

19. Gaskin, *Ina May's Guide*.

20. Gaskin, *Ina May's Guide*.

21. Gaskin, *Ina May's Guide*.

22. Sarah J. Buckley, *Gentle Birth, Gentle Mothering: The Wisdom and Science of Gentle Choices in Pregnancy, Birth, and Parenting*. (Brisbane: One Moon Press, 2005).

23. Gaskin, *Ina May's Guide*.

24. Gaskin, *Ina May's Guide*.

25. Gaskin, *Ina May's Guide*.

26. Gaskin, *Ina May's Guide.*

27. Gaskin, *Ina May's Guide.*

28. Cheryl Mutch, "Weaning from the Breast." *National Center for Biotechnology Information.* Canadian Paediatric Society. (April 2004). DOI: 10.1093/pch/9.4.249.

29. Gaskin, *Ina May's Guide.*

Chapter 6

1. "Infant and Young Child Feeding." *World Health Organization.* (June 9, 2021). https://www.who.int/news-room/fact-sheets/detail/infant-and-young-child-feeding.

2. "Infant Food and Feeding." *American Academy of Pediatrics.* (Accessed June 26, 2021). https://www.aap.org/en-us/advocacy-and-policy/aap-health-initiatives/HALF-Implementation-Guide/Age-Specific-Content/Pages/Infant-Food-and-Feeding.aspx.

3. Jenna Helwig, *Baby-Led Feeding: A Natural Way to Raise Happy, Independent Eaters.* (Boston: Houghton Mifflin Harcourt, 2018).

4. Malina Malkani, *Simple & Safe Baby-Led Weaning: How to Integrate Foods, Master Portion Sizes, and Identify Allergies.* (Emeryville: Rockridge Press, 2020).

5. Gill Rapley and Tracey Murkett. *Baby-Led Weaning: The Essential Guide to Introducing Solid Foods-and Helping Your Baby to Grow Up a Happy and Confident Eater.* (New York: Experiment, 2010).

6. Helwig, *Baby-Led Feeding.*

7. Helwig, *Baby-Led Feeding.*

8. Malkani, *Simple & Safe.*

9. Malkani, *Simple & Safe.*

10. Malkani, *Simple & Safe.*

11. Malkani, *Simple & Safe*.

12. Malkani, *Simple & Safe*.

13. Helwig, *Baby-Led Feeding*.

14. Helwig, *Baby-Led Feeding*.

15. Malkani, *Simple & Safe*.

16. Malkani, *Simple & Safe*.

17. Giulia Enders, *Gut: The Inside Story of Our Body's Most Underrated Organ*. (New York: Greystone Books, 2015).

18. "Constipation in Children." *Mayo Clinic*. Mayo Foundation for Medical Education and Research. (August 6, 2019). https://www.mayoclinic.org/diseases-conditions/constipation-in-children/symptoms-causes/syc-20354242.

19. "Sodium and Potassium Dietary Reference Intake Values Updated in New Report; Introduces New Category for Sodium Based on Chronic Disease Risk Reduction." *The National Academies of Sciences, Engineering, Medicine*. (March 5, 2019). https://www.nationalacademies.org/news/2019/03/sodium-and-potassium-dietary-reference-intake-values-updated-in-new-report.

20. Malkani, *Simple & Safe*.

21. Malkani, *Simple & Safe*.

Chapter 7

1. Jennifer Margulis, *The Business of Baby: What Doctors Don't Tell You, What Corporations Try to Sell You, and How to Put Your Pregnancy, Childbirth, and Baby Before Their Bottom Line*. (New York: Scribner, 2013).

2. Yekaterina Chzhen, Anna Gromada, and Gwyther Rees. "Are the World's Richest Countries Family Friendly? Policy in the OECD and EU." *Unicef*. Unicef, Office of Research. (June. 2019). https://www.unicef-irc.org/publications/pdf/Family-Friendly-Policies-Research_UNICEF_%202019.pdf.

3. Matt Turner, "Here's How Much Paid Leave New Mothers and Fathers Get in 11 Different Countries." *Business Insider.* (September 7, 2017). https://www.businessinsider.com/maternity-leave-worldwide-2017-8#italy-every-mother-gets-at-least-five-months-maternity-leave-9.

4. Lynda Laughlin, "Maternity Leave and Employment Patterns of First-Time Mothers: 1961–2008." *U.S. Census Bureau.* Economics and Statistics Administration. (October 2011). https://www.census.gov/prod/2011pubs/p70-128.pdf.

5. Julie Sullivan, "Comparing Characteristics and Selected Expenditures of Dual- and Single-Income Households with Children." *U.S. Bureau of Labor Statistics.* (September 2020). https://www.bls.gov/opub/mlr/2020/article/comparing-characteristics-and-selected-expenditures-of-dual-and-single-income-households-with-children.htm.

6. George Wootan, "Mother-Baby Separation." *The Natural Child Project.* (Accessed June 26, 2021). https://www.naturalchild.org/articles/guest/george_wootan2.html.

7. Wooten, "Mother-Baby Separation."

Chapter 8

1. "Media and Young Minds." *American Academy of Pediatrics.* 138, no. 5 (November 1, 2016). DOI: 10.1542/peds.2016-2591.

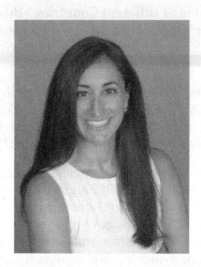

Laura Rafferty lives in upstate New York with her husband, Justin, and her son, Jack. It's a perfect place to live for her, as she loves all four seasons and all of the corresponding outdoor activities.

Her favorite things to do are running, traveling, cooking and reading. Laura has worked in corporate America for her entire career but writing a book has been one of her lifelong dreams.

Becoming a mother gave her the content and the motivation to make that dream a reality. As an avid reader, research for the book was more of a hobby than a chore. And she shared her journey in the book to give other mamas the support and sanity check that she was looking for!

Made in the USA
Middletown, DE
06 April 2023